1,137 Secrets for **living well** with DIABETES

ALSO BY JUDITH H. MCQUOWN

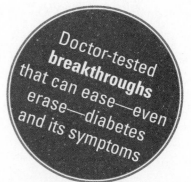

Doctor-tested **breakthroughs** that can ease—even erase—diabetes and its symptoms

1,137

Secrets for **living well** with

DIABETES

Judith H. McQuown

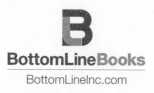

BottomLineBooks

BottomLineInc.com

Every area of trouble gives out a ray of hope, and the one unchangeable certainty is that nothing is certain or unchangeable.
— *John F. Kennedy*

What would life be if we had no courage to attempt anything?
— *Vincent van Gogh*

When you're going through hell, keep going.
—*Winston Churchill*

For

Harold Allen Lightman

Contents

CHAPTER 2

Weight Loss and Nutrition

Contents

CHAPTER 3

Working with Your Doctors and Other Health-Care Professionals

CHAPTER 4

Avoiding/Surviving Hospitals and Emergency Rooms

Contents

CHAPTER 5

Exercise

CHAPTER 6

Dealing with Depression and Stress

CHAPTER 7

Tips for Children with Diabetes and Their Parents

CHAPTER 8

Tips for Diabetics Who Live Alone

Thinking Clearly

Eyes

Cardiovascular

Foreword

by Ronald Tamler, MD, PhD, MB, CNSC, COE

Through the crackle of sound waves that had been compressed over and over into tiny data packets to transmit information efficiently, the worry and anguish in my friend's words were as crystal-clear as if he were standing right next to me: He had found his baby daughter, just nine months old, barely breathing and dehydrated. A finger stick in the ER brought certainty: Blood glucose 600. Ketones. ICU.

Diagnosis: Diabetes.

What would become of her? Would she have a life?

The first question was answered easily over the next few days. Although diabetic ketoacidosis—the metabolic emergency that stems from not making or getting enough insulin—is still a life-threatening condition with a mortality rate of up to 10%, the young parents had gotten their daughter help in time. But as they were absorbing information about finger sticks, insulin dosing and pharmacology, hypoglycemia and sick days, the second question remained. Would their young daughter have a life? Friends and relatives were calling with grave stories they had heard: Legs amputated, dialysis, hypoglycemic coma. Doom!

We cure appendicitis. We mend a broken bone. We manage diabetes. "How's life?"

"I manage."

Does this sound like thriving? Living with diabetes is a full-time job with no immediate payoff. Would my friend's baby daughter manage? Would she be exposed to ridicule and discrimination from ill-informed friends or future employers who think that diabetes is a condition people bring on themselves as the result of a gluttonous lifestyle?

I knew my friend would soon get bombarded with well-meaning bits of news: Cell cultures making insulin. Worms exposed to a drug and cured of diabetes. And—of course—myriad mice that were thriving on one kind of diabetes treatment or another. I advised him to ignore all of these things. Instead, I sent him a list of famous and successful people with type 1 (formerly called "juvenile") diabetes. My friend's baby daughter would not be held back and could become a Supreme Court justice, or a rock star, or an athlete.

On the phone that desperate night, I told him the story of a patient of mine: In 2007, I met a vigorous 66-year-old lady with volatile ("brittle") type 1 diabetes. The only thing reliable about her blood glucose was its inverse relation to the stock market. Yet she had persisted—no, thrived—building a career, staving off complications, living through technological advances over the course of over three decades with diabetes. You guessed it: That patient is none other than Judith McQuown.

During her first visit with me, she demanded, "Just get me to 90. That's a pretty good age."

OK, I'm up for the challenge, I thought.

Over the next 10 years, I accompanied her on her journey, an adviser to a rather stubborn and creative captain of her own ship.

When Judith turned seventy-five, I congratulated her and expected something like an "attaboy!" Instead, she replied, "Ninety looks so close now. I think 120 sounds a lot better!"

And while Judith is a special person, I have many patients who have had diabetes for 30, 40, 50, or 60 years and live full, normal lives.

These folks have witnessed the incremental evolution of diabetes diagnostics and therapeutics. Nobody has to guess their blood glucose after urinating on a stick anymore. Nobody has to inject insulin from a pig or a cow every four hours in order to survive. Instead, we now have drugs that help people with type 2 diabetes make more insulin—but only if the body needs it. Drugs that help obese people with diabetes lose weight. Drugs that make people urinate extra sugar and may drastically cut down on heart disease. Small pumps that can be programmed to deliver a different dose of insulin at different times of day (less if you are exercising, more if you eat a bowl of pasta), and continuous glucose monitors that can assess blood-glucose trends and sound the alarm fairly reliably when blood-glucose levels are out of bounds. We are about to take the next step in that evolution, as the first "closed-loop" systems are getting ready to hit the market. A sensor continuously telling a device running an algorithm checking the blood glucose, and the algorithm telling an insulin pump how much insulin to deliver. No human intervention required, or desired—we'd just mess it up anyway.

Ultimately, though, good diabetes management is not rocket science or brain surgery. (Frankly, you should probably decline politely if either offers to manage your diabetes.) Every reasonably good medical student knows what goes into preventing diabetes complications.

Keep your blood sugar reasonably controlled. Avoid low blood sugars. Take a (generic) blood pressure medication to help prevent kidney disease. Take a (generic) statin drug to lower cholesterol. Live a healthful life to decrease your medication load. Don't smoke. Examine your feet. See your eye doctor twice a year. We have known this for decades. But for one reason or another, be it education, finances, or the fatigue that comes from dealing with a chronic condition every single day of one's life, only a small minority of people with diabetes are taking all these steps that, taken together, massively lower the risk of complications and death from diabetes.

When my friend heard of Judith's story, how she rejected her target life expectancy, he knew that diabetes would not hold back his little girl. Within a few weeks, she was on an insulin pump, and the family had connected online with others in a similar situation, providing each other with advice and support. At work now, Mommy's phone beeps when her two-year-old has abnormal blood glucose miles away in day care.

Everybody has moments in which the challenges of diabetes seem overwhelming. So many questions, so much to learn, so much to keep track of! Thank goodness Judith McQuown has made it her mission to live to tell the story with a different kind of diabetes book. If only one of these 1,137 "secret tips" helps you to live well with diabetes, it will have fulfilled its purpose.

Read it in good health!

—Ronald Tamler, MD, PhD, MB, CNSC, COE
Clinical Director, Mount Sinai Diabetes Center
Associate Professor of Medicine,
Division of Endocrinology, Diabetes & Bone Disease,
Mount Sinai School of Medicine

Introduction

I was diagnosed as a type 2 diabetic thirty years ago, in 1987, although I had probably had diabetes for two or three years at that point. After a six-month "honeymoon" on oral hypoglycemics (pills that lower blood glucose) I had to be switched to insulin. I have now been injecting insulin for 30 years.

Thanks to the advances in diabetes research over the past 30 years, I now know that it is probable that I had type 1.5 diabetes, also known as LADA (Latent Autoimmune Diabetes in Adults or Slow-Onset type 1). I don't think that it makes much difference now. We can't change the past. But we can make changes now to improve our health.

In the 30 years that I have had diabetes, I have learned many things. The two most important have been (1) to keep learning about this chronic disease because there have been and will be so many advances in research and treatment, and (2) to always have a sense of humor and a "Plan B" so that life's little curves and uncertainties don't create stress.

In those 30 years, my endocrinologists have changed my medications many times. My insulin syringes and needle sizes have gotten smaller. My oral medications have changed, and now I am off them completely. With all these changes, my fasting blood glucose is now normal, although I need insulin to keep it there. My other readings are within range. I am a very happy woman!

This is a book full of hope and practicality. This is a book with hundreds of ideas you can use to live well despite your diabetes. You probably know that diabetes is now classified as a pandemic (worldwide epidemic). It even landed a *Time* magazine cover story in January 2016.

The statistics are staggering. According to the World Health Organization, 422 million people had diabetes in 2014, and type 2 diabetes has quadrupled in the past 40 years. Industrialization is not bringing good health along with it. It is projected that by 2030, 360 million residents of China and more than 79 million in India will have diabetes. More than 14 million residents of Mexico have diabetes, and the number is certain to increase. No surprise—over 50 million adults there

1

are overweight or obese. That's the reason for Mexico's "soda tax," which increases the price of sugary drinks by 10% and the price of junk food by 8%. Thirty-seven million Latin Americans are diabetic, and the World Bank predicts that this number will surge to 57 million by 2030. In Saudi Arabia, according to a May 3, 2016, article in *Al Arabiya*, 72% of the population is overweight or obese—44% of women and 26.4% of men. In Israel, 70% of the men and 65% of women aged 45-64 are overweight or obese.

Most worldwide diabetes sufferers have type 2 diabetes, which is associated with obesity and inactivity. Obesity affects three times as many people in the United Kingdom as it did 20 years ago. A 2013 survey found that 67% of men and 57% of women were overweight or obese as defined by their BMI. *These grim statistics could lead to the first drop in British life expectancy in over a century because obesity shortens people's lives.* The more you weigh, the more likely you are to die young.

In the United States, there are close to 30 million people estimated to have diabetes, with more than 1.2 million new cases diagnosed in 2015. Of the total, more than eight million were undiagnosed. Of the 30 million, close to 4 million are African-American, more than double the 2.7 million in 2003; 0.8 million are Native Americans living on reservations—a staggering eightfold increase—and some Indian nations have a 50% diabetes rate. Over 13.4 million are women, and 10.5 million are senior citizens. (Obviously, some people with diabetes belong to two or three of these categories.)

In 2014, the U.S. Department of Agriculture reported that the average American consumes more than 150 pounds of refined sugar per year. For every health-conscious American who eats only five pounds of sugar per year, there is one who consumes more than 295 pounds per year. That may explain the success of Lifetime-TV's *My 600-Pound Life*.

In response to the diabetes pandemic, in June 2016, Philadelphia became the first major U.S. city to enact a "sugar drink" tax amounting to 1.5 cents per ounce, or 48 cents per quart. In November 2016, San Francisco, Oakland, and many other Bay Area governments approved a sugary drink tax of one cent per ounce, or 32 cents per quart. And in June 2017, Seattle also passed a sugary beverage tax of 1.75 cents per ounce, or 56 cents per quart.

Countless millions more have started down the ugly road to diabetes. Known variously as "metabolic syndrome" or "Syndrome X," this condition is defined by the National Institutes of Health as a person's having at least three out of five of the following symptoms…

- **Heavy abdominal fat, with a waistline over 40 inches for men, over 35 inches for women**

- **Blood pressure higher than 130/85**

- **HDL (good) cholesterol lower than 40 mg/dL**

- Triglycerides greater than or equal to 150 mg/dL

- Fasting blood glucose greater than or equal to 110 mg/dL

At least 113 million American adults—more than 35% of the population—have metabolic syndrome, which affects more than 45% of Americans in their 60s and 70s.

"Prediabetes" is another condition that leads to full-blown diabetes if left unchecked. An estimated 86 million Americans have this condition, which is identified by a fasting blood-glucose level higher than 100 mg/dL. Unless they lose weight and start exercising, 15% to 30% will develop full-blown type 2 diabetes within five years.

The tips in this book are designed to help people with prediabetes, too. With a little care, self-discipline, and good medical treatment, they will be able to avoid or postpone the onset of diabetes and to minimize its potential damage.

The Cost of Diabetes

The annual economic cost of diabetes in 2014 was $322 billion, up from $245 billion in 2012, only two years earlier. This represents a huge chunk of every health-care dollar spent in the United States. Many experts fear that diabetes' annual costs could bankrupt Social Security by 2025.

Ever wondered why? Let's examine some scary statistics:

The average American consumes more than 150 pounds of sugar per year. (Yes, it bears repeating!)

Over 30% of all vegetables eaten in the United States are French fries. This does not include potato chips and other potato snacks.

What Americans spend on fast food has risen to $1,300 per person per year, about $420 billion total.

As a result, today's American children may be the first modern generation to have shorter life expectancies than their parents.

Today's Battle of the Bulge is far more lethal than the one we fought and won more than 70 years ago. That World War II battle suffered more than 180,000 casualties in six weeks of fighting. This battle is ongoing and will result in millions of diabetes-related deaths in the next decade alone. Both type 2s, who often battle overweight and obesity, and type 1s, who may not have weight problems, are at risk and must plan for their healthy futures.

Think of your diabetes as a time bomb with a very long fuse. It's a time bomb because eventually it could causer heart disease, stroke, kidney disease, blindness, and some forms of cancer. But its long fuse means that you can take action to prevent or delay those deadly diseases and live a long, happy, and productive life.

The tips in these chapters come from many sources: Friends, friends of friends all over the United States, parents and teachers of children with diabetes, doctors and researchers, a diabetes support group in New York City, and many people I met online. And many of these tips are my own, based on hard-earned personal experience. While these tips have been reviewed by medical professionals, check with your own doctors because diabetes is a very individual disease.

The tips in these chapters may seem to be random. That's because I want you to read each one separately and think about it for a minute or two. In that way, the tips will be of the greatest help to you and your family. You will notice that nearly half the tips are concentrated in two chapters: "Weight Loss and Nutrition" and "Dealing with Depression and Stress." That is because I believe that if you lose weight, eat more healthfully, and overcome depression and stress at least half the time, you will manage your diabetes successfully. Consult the index in this edition if you are looking for a specific topic.

I have not included any tips about insulin pumps because these marvelous machines have already been covered exhaustively in Gabrielle Kaplan-Mayer's *excellent* book, *Insulin Pump Therapy Demystified* (revised edition 2013). Even in this area there have been recent radical changes. In April 2016, NPR Radio station WNYC reported that Dana Lewis, a type 1 diabetic who was dissatisfied with her insulin pump's shortcomings, hacked together her own artificial pancreas. Now, more than 50 individuals with type 1 have built versions of Dana's system, OpenAPS (Open Artificial Pancreas System), thanks to Ben West, a brilliant San Francisco software engineer and type 1 diabetic. West was the first to write the essential code that lets type 1s hack their insulin pumps to improve their functioning. These "hackathons" are increasing, to the delight of their participants.

And now here's the most important tip...

1 Be creative!

Regard diabetes as a challenging disease you can outsmart. Think outside the box to solve problems and achieve results.

It's up to you—and these tips will help!

CHAPTER 1

Drugs and Equipment

2 Know that no drug works for everyone...

Every patient is a unique individual. Not only does no drug work for everyone, but it is very likely that, as time passes, your body will get used to a drug you are taking, or your condition will change (or both), and you will have to change the dosage of the drug or even switch to another drug. Fortunately, there are many drugs for the treatment of diabetes—and even more in the pipeline—so your doctor's changing them shouldn't be a problem.

3 ...And that many drugs take getting used to.

When your doctor gives you a new or different drug, or a new dosage or formulation, it may take several days to a week for your body to get used to it and for it to work well.

If you have an adverse reaction, call your doctor immediately. Otherwise, give the drug a chance to work.

4 Be aware that weight loss can lower your drug requirements.

Even if you've lost only 10 or 15 pounds, you may need to have your medication changed. Call your doctor, especially if you start having two or three low blood-glucose readings per week.

5 Test often.

If you use insulin, you should be testing your blood glucose at least three or four times a day. Most of us long-timers on insulin test more than five times a day, always before meals, before and after exercise, and before bed. If you're not on insulin, you might be tempted to test less frequently—some diabetics test once a day or less—but the more often you test, the more precise information you have about your blood-glucose numbers, and the better care you can take of yourself.

Test-strip suppliers—usually connected with insurance providers—will generally give you only five or six test strips a day—500 for a three-month period. But they don't always tell you that you can get more without having to pay for them.

All you need is a doctor's prescription with the magic words "medical necessity," the number of times a day you test, and the total number of strips you need for the allotted time period, often three months. Doctors and insurance providers are usually happy to do this because they know that the more frequently you test, the less likely it is that you will develop expensive diabetic complications.

6 Minimize the sticking point.

If you test your blood glucose with a lancet several times a day, in time your fingertips will resemble a pincushion. Insulin users can minimize these holes by using the needle from their last insulin syringe, after wiping it with an alcohol swab to sterilize it. The needle is much thinner, so it inflicts less damage to your tissues—and less pain.

However, my friend Mischa, who is much taller and outweighs me by over 100 pounds, argues that a lancet has a major advantage for the squeamish. *It* does the work, rather than your having to do the finger sticks yourself.

Choose the instrument and method that makes you feel the most comfortable. When insulin needles are

Photo: Simpson33

thinner than lancets, you may prefer doing finger sticks with them. When newer, thinner lancets are available, you may want to switch—and use them with or without the lancing device.

7 Practice syringe smarts.

As syringe needles have become progressively shorter and thinner, I have changed sizes three or four times in the past 10 years. Thinner, shorter needles cause less tissue damage and are less painful. Pharmacists and manufacturers' websites as well as physicians are excellent sources of what's new.

8 Beware: Your insulin pump can be hacked (but it probably won't be).

On October 4, 2016, CNBC reported that Johnson & Johnson's One Touch Ping insulin pump had been hacked into, putting at risk more than 114,000 patients, with the possibility of changing their insulin dosage. Rapid7 researcher and security consultant Jay Radcliffe, himself a diabetic, hacked into his own insulin pump to show how this hacking could be done. He pointed out to CNBC viewers that hackers would have to be within 25 feet of the insulin pump they wanted to disable in order to turn off the radio frequency connected to the pump. While theoretically possible, this scenario is not likely, and probably belongs in a spy novel or film script.

9 Double up on your insulin.

Until Murphy's Law is repealed, the one time a year that you drop a bottle of insulin and break it is during a three-day blizzard.

Remember the Boy Scout motto and be prepared. This prevents panic and emergencies.

Always make sure that you have at least two bottles of every type of insulin you are taking. Most insurance plans will send you a three-month supply of each insulin you take, but if they give you a hard time, just ask your doctor to write "medical necessity" on the prescription.

10 Try this modified 72-hour test.

The 72-hour blood-glucose test is a useful tool for diagnosing when, how, and why some diabetic patients experience gyrating blood-glucose levels for no apparent reason, a condition known as "brittle diabetes."

The results of this test may help you get a continuous glucose monitor (CGM) from your insurance provider if your doctor thinks it is warranted and may help you. (See Tip 11 for details.)

A physician or nurse inserts a tiny sensor into your abdomen and tapes it securely. It takes minute blood samples every five minutes and transmits them to a monitor clipped onto your waistband or underwear (or pajamas when you're asleep). The monitor registers these 864 blood-glucose readings, which are downloaded to a computer and analyzed at the end of 72 hours. During the test, ERROR messages and beeps will alert you to problems.

Unfortunately, this equipment can malfunction, and then the test will have to be aborted. A company representative told me that this happens a little more than 10% of the time. (My estimate is closer to 20% after two of my tests in two months with different sensors and monitors had to be aborted.)

Undeterred, I decided to create a modified test. I urge you to try it, too, if your monitor malfunctions, or if your insurance does not cover the test.

Choose a three-day weekend, or three consecutive days when you can work from home. Do finger sticks every hour on the hour (or as close to it as you can) from the time you wake up until bedtime and, if possible, at least once during the middle of the night. Keep a detailed log of your readings. Also log in your insulin dosages, other medication, meals, exercise, and hypoglycemic "events." Your goal is to have at least 45 blood-glucose readings over three days. Admittedly, it's a lot of work, but it's only three days, and the results, once analyzed by your doctor, will give you better control of your diabetes.

Why do this at home? Some critics of this strategy feel that doing this test during three consecutive days in the workplace/office produces more accurate results. However, other medical professionals believe that testing your blood glucose every hour on the hour while at your job could create so much stress that the blood-glucose numbers would be high and therefore inaccurate. It's a very individual decision, but I'll vote with the second group.

11 Be aware that CGMs are now covered under Medicare Part B.

In mid-January 2017, the Centers for Medicare & Medicaid Services ruled that continuous glucose monitors (CGMs) would be regarded as durable medical equipment covered under Medicare Part B. This action has taken a long time to finalize and many patients with diabetes will benefit from it.

12 Know when half-measures work best.

Although this tip seems obvious, few doctors suggest it. Often—especially in newly diagnosed type 1 (insulin-dependent) diabetics—10 (or any whole number of insulin units) is too little, but 11 is too much.

Syringes are designed with enough space between units to get midpoints, so you can measure 10 ½ units pretty accurately. With your doctor's approval, try the half-unit dosage for at least three days and see if your results improve. And now some insulin pens are calibrated in half-units too!

13 Watch when pills work too quickly.

Similarly, in some individuals with diabetes, oral hypoglycemics can kick in too quickly, causing rapid drops in blood glucose. For a slower, smoother evening out, ask your doctor whether a time-release oral hypoglycemic would work better for you.

14 Note post-9/11 travel rules.

Official policy: Increased security since September 11, 2001, means that you will have to prove that your syringes, insulin, blood-glucose meter, test strips, glucagon, and other gear are for your diabetes and that it is medically necessary for you to carry them. If you are wearing an insulin pump, you will have to show that to airport security, too.

You need a letter from your doctor stating that you have diabetes and that you need to carry all these drugs and equipment. Most important, you will need to carry your insulin in the prescription box it came in, and at least one *unopened* package of syringes, as well as the syringes you need, so that airport security can verify that your loose syringes are identical to the packaged ones.

Although this is the official policy, it does not seem enforced consistently or as strongly as these paragraphs suggest. Many travelers with diabetes have never had their drugs or diabetes supplies questioned and have never been asked to produce a letter from their doctor.

15 Familiarize yourself with Lantus: The "Poor Patient's Pump."

Long-acting insulin Lantus is a godsend for many diabetic patients whose blood glucose yo-yo'd on Ultralente and other long-acting insulins. Because Lantus has a duration of approximately 24 hours, it provides a basal level that mimics the action of a normal pancreas, or of a pump that releases small doses of insulin continuously.

With Lantus, you will still have to use a fast-acting insulin, like Humalog or NovaLog to cover your meals, and you will have to use *separate* syringes for Lantus and the fast-acting insulin because they react with each other. However, if Lantus gives you better blood-glucose control, you may be able to skip or reduce your before-lunch or before-dinner Humalog.

For newer, longer-acting insulins approved by the FDA from 2013 to 2017, read the tips at the end of this chapter.

16 "My diabetes isn't serious because I'm only taking pills" is a myth.

Many patients with type 2 diabetes don't take their disease seriously enough. They say, "My diabetes isn't serious because I don't have to take insulin. I'm only taking pills."

And then, because it isn't "serious," they act as if they don't have diabetes at all: They don't test their blood glucose and they don't watch their calorie or carbohydrate consumption. Many type 2s are overweight or even clinically obese, but make no attempt to diet.

Over the years, this cavalier attitude causes serious, irreversible damage, like neuropathy, retina problems, and gangrene. One of my type 2 "non-insulin-dependent" friends who disregarded diet and exercise for years is waiting for a kidney transplant and will likely need dialysis before then. Both are painful, difficult, life-threatening options.

How you take care of yourself *now* is an investment in your healthy *future*.

17 Starting insulin therapy immediately may be a smart move.

You are newly diagnosed with type 2 diabetes, which means that your pancreas is still making insulin. But your doctor recommends insulin injections anyway. How come?

Recent research suggests that many new type 2s are stressing their pancreases in the early days of their disease. That's why there is often a "honeymoon" of several months to a year when oral medications work, followed by an inevitable burnout, when their pancreases stop manufacturing insulin. At that point, they must take insulin for the rest of their lives.

However, if you are put on insulin immediately, your overburdened pancreas is able to rest and recuperate. Later—especially if you are able to go from obese to overweight, or overweight to normal weight—you may be able to switch from insulin to pills.

Research published in February 2015 in *The Lancet Diabetes & Endocrinology* reported several studies that focused on the temporary use of insulin to restore glucose control in patients with type 2 diabetes: "The results showed that a two- to five-week course of short-term intensive insulin therapy (IIT) can induce remission in patients who are early in the course of type 2 diabetes. At three months after stopping the IIT, 66% of patients were still in remission, and at six months, 59% were still in remission."

These results are amazing!

18 Timing your Lantus can make a big difference.

Timing your Lantus (or other very-long-acting insulin) when you wake up rather than before bedtime seems to control blood glucose better. Much of the evidence is anecdotal, but many insulin-dependent diabetics have experienced these results. It's certainly worth discussing with your doctor.

19 Double-check if your results look strange.

Every so often, you'll get a blood-glucose result that looks strange. It's way too high or too low, but you don't feel any different.

Before adjusting your medication or popping some glucose tablets, double-check. First, make sure that the area you're taking blood from is absolutely clean. Fingertips especially can pick up trace amounts of food or other substances that can distort your test results.

Then make sure that the sample is really all blood—not half blood and half clear fluid (serum), which can happen in cold weather. See that it fills the test chamber completely. (Most meters will show an ERROR message if there's a problem with your sample.)

If this test is substantially different from the first, repeat the test a third time. The second and third tests should show similar readings. Use an average of these two readings to get a fairly accurate test result.

20 Keep a glucagon kit. It can save your life.

If you have ever fainted from severe hypoglycemia (or come close), you *must* keep a glucagon kit handy for future emergencies when you are unable to swallow.

Glucagon is a hormone that raises your blood sugar by increasing the rate at which glycogen, which is stored in the liver, breaks down and is converted into glucose. It works very quickly.

Since preparing and injecting the glucagon is a little complex, have one or more family members or close friends familiarize themselves with the kit and its instructions. They should also practice by giving you your insulin shot now and then.

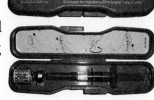

Photo: Bing/Eli Lilly

It is imperative that your designated "medic" act quickly. The longer you are unconscious, the more dangerous it is. Brain damage can start in 30 minutes!

Note: Sometimes two injections are needed, so you may want to keep two kits on hand. Fortunately, they can be kept at room temperature, and they have a shelf life of 18 months.

Unfortunately, glucagon kits are useless if you live alone. When your blood glucose drops to 30 or 40, you are too uncoordinated to mix the glucagon and inject it. If you even suspect that your blood glucose is tanking, jam a tube of glucose gel into your mouth and swallow it or put some glucose tablets into your mouth and swallow them quickly.

21 Participate in a clinical trial.

Most clinical trials for promising new drugs are for Phase II (efficacy), Phase III (the new drug vs. drugs already in use or vs. a standard treatment), or a combined Phase II/III study.

These drugs have already passed Phase I (safety) trials and have been approved by the FDA for further study.

When you volunteer for a clinical trial, there is a possibility that you will receive the placebo (inert drug) rather than the new drug. In fact, in double-blind studies, which are the most common type, the researchers do not know which patients are getting the new drug and which the placebo.

In either case, however, you should receive superb medical care from some of the most talented and attentive doctors and researchers in the country. And you may help with the discovery of a miraculous new drug!

22 Replace your insulin frequently.

Remember these guidelines to keep your insulin potent…

●**An unopened vial stored in the refrigerator should last until the expiration date.** However, just to make sure, start using it at least two months before the expiration date.

●**An unopened vial stored at room temperature lasts 28 days.**

●**An opened vial stored in the refrigerator lasts 28 days.**

●**An opened vial stored at room temperature lasts 28 days.**

23 Choose sugar-free medications.

Many over-the-counter medications, like cough syrups and antacids, contain sugars like high-fructose corn syrup, which create a problem in controlling your blood glucose.

Read labels carefully. Choose medicines that display "sugar-free" wording prominently, although they may be more expensive. Ask your doctor or pharmacist for advice.

24 Ask about statins.

Diabetes is a serious risk for heart disease. And multiple studies have shown that statins can cut the risk of heart disease and stroke in people with diabetes by about one-third. Unfortunately, statins are underprescribed for women.

According to a May 5, 2016, study by Boston's Brigham and Women's Hospital published in *PLOS ONE*, four factors may account for differences between statin prescribing for men and women with coronary artery disease (CAD)—evaluation by a cardiologist, history of reported adverse reaction to statins, patient age, and smoking history.

As CAD in women often has no symptoms, it's a good idea to consult a cardiologist and ask about a statin prescription. On the other hand, statins can cause serious side effects in postmenopausal women, so be sure to discuss with your doctor if the benefits of statin medication outweigh the risks.

25 Gauge size makes a big difference.

Needle and lancet sizes are stated in wire gauge, whose numbers look pretty close together: 28, 30, 31, 33 gauge. But there's a big difference.

GAUGE SIZE	MILLIMETERS
28	0.32
30	0.25
31	0.22
33	0.18

Note that as the gauge increases, the size in millimeters decreases.

A little quick arithmetic shows you that a 33-gauge lancet is 28% smaller than a 30-gauge lancet, and a 31-gauge syringe needle is 12% smaller than a 30-gauge syringe needle. Your fingers (and other test spots) and insulin injection sites will definitely notice the difference—less pain and less tissue damage.

26 Avoid prescription errors.

With the advent of FDA-mandated emailed prescriptions, doctors' illegible handwriting may be a thing of the distant, jokey past.

Not so fast! To avoid errors in your prescriptions, ask your doctor to spell out the name of the medication and write it down, along with the correct dosage and time(s) you should take it. When you pick up the prescription, compare the label with your notes.

You can minimize the chance of errors even more by getting your prescription filled in the early afternoon, the slowest time of the day, when pharmacist mistakes are the least likely.

And make sure that the contents of your filled prescription are correct. Just last month, only half my boxes of blood glucose test strips were correct. Half were for another meter model and had to be returned.

27 Check out pill splitters and cut your drug bills in half.

This strategy works best (a) when your drug plan has a flat copayment per drug per month regardless of the dosage; (b) your medication is a pill that comes in several dosages; (c) your doctor is willing to write a prescription for pills that are double your dosage and tells you that it is OK for you to split these pills in half.

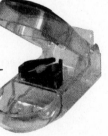

Buy a pill splitter at your pharmacy—it should cost about $3 to $5. Then follow the directions to cut a pill in half, take half (this is your regular dosage), and wrap the other half in plastic for your next dose. Doing this will turn one month's supply into two, thus cutting your drug bill in half.

Photo: 21bgil

28 Keep antibiotics handy.

Do you catch the same kind of "bug" every year? Like strep throat? Does your doctor prescribe the same antibiotic? Then it's a good idea to start taking that antibiotic quickly to prevent a long, serious illness that might lead to hospitalization. One savvy diabetic friend and her doctor agreed on this game plan so that she can start treatment immediately.

Her doctor gives her a prescription for 10 days' worth of an antibiotic that she has taken successfully for many years, and she fills it and stores it away.

When she gets sick, she takes aspirin, vitamin C , and chicken soup loaded with garlic for two or three days. Then she calls her doctor to make sure her symptoms sound like those of a bacterial infection. If her doctor gives her the OK, she starts the antibiotic without risking exposure to other "bugs" in his waiting room.

But if she is still sick after two or three days on the antibiotic, she *must* call her doctor and come in for an examination and lab tests.

This treatment strategy has worked so well that she has fought the bug and avoided serious complications for many years—all by having her antibiotics within arm's reach.

29 Use antibiotics correctly to keep superbugs away.

In a June 3, 2016, CNBC interview, Center for American Progress Fellow Ezekiel Emanuel, MD, pointed out that in the past few years, superbugs—antibiotic-resistant bacteria—have received tremendous press coverage because they have caused so many patient deaths. *These microscopic monsters have grown in power and ferocity due to two major causes…*

1. Many doctors overprescribe and misprescribe antibiotics. These drugs work only against bacterial infections, not viral infections. When antibiotics are used for the wrong diseases, they don't kill anything. They create superbugs.

2. Many patients do not take the full course of their antibiotics. Instead of taking the full 10-day dose, they take their antibiotics for three or four days and feel better, so they quit taking the drug. After all, they're better, aren't they? What's the result? Surviving superbugs are more powerful, and they multiply and are able to fight more antibiotics.

30 Investigate "flexible" insulin.

In a perfect world, we would start eating a meal between 30 and 45 minutes after injecting insulin.

But in the real world, we might inject insulin, go to a restaurant or dinner party, order, and then wait and wait as our blood glucose drops, in the certain knowledge that the insulin and our food will not coincide.

Humalog and other new insulins discussed in the tips at the end of this chapter are faster-acting and more flexible. Not only can they be injected just before you eat, they can also be injected immediately after you eat. In fact, you might even think of these insulins as "oops!" or morning-after drugs because if you overeat at dinner or at a party, you can increase your dosage anywhere from immediately after to the next morning to compensate for the extra carbohydrates.

31 Don't blame yourself if you need to increase your dosage.

After being on a medication for some time, the human body often stops responding to it as effectively as it used to. We need more of it—or maybe even a different drug—to achieve the desired result.

Don't blame yourself. It happens all the time and there's nothing you can do about it—just ask your doctor or pharmacist.

32 Ask: How long will it take?

When your doctor prescribes a new drug, ask how long it will take for you to see results. This is almost as important as asking about side effects.

33 Ask your doctor these three questions at every appointment.

It's tempting for both patients and their doctors to continue on the same medications year after year, but this may not be the smartest strategy. *Always ask your doctor...*

- **Do I still need this drug?**
- **Are there newer/better drugs that I can substitute?**
- **If I stay on this drug, is my current dose still proper?**

34 Evaluate your diet with every new medication.

When your doctor prescribes a new drug, always ask whether there are foods you should avoid.

Many of us know that grapefruit and grapefruit juice can interact dangerously with more than 50 drugs (such as statins, which lower cholesterol, and hypertension medications).

But potassium-rich bananas can also react badly with ACE inhibitors, which are taken for high blood pressure and congestive heart failure, producing a double whammy in potassium levels, which can result in irregular heartbeats and palpitations.

35 Update your immunizations.

You need diphtheria and tetanus booster shots every 10 years. If you don't remember the last time you had a booster shot, it's probably time to get one. Many people with diabetes don't have the same doctors they had 10 years ago, and they may not keep good records. For more information, contact Immunization Action Coalition at (651) 647-9009 or log on to Immunize.org.

36 Get your flu shot early in the morning.

A University of Birmingham (UK) study, published in *Vaccine* in April 2016, found that older adults who got a flu shot in the morning had four times as many antibodies fighting swine flu and 50% more against influenza B than those who got an afternoon shot. That's a lot of extra protection!

37 Ask your doctor about two flu shots.

A 2015 Centers for Disease Control and Prevention (CDC) report recommends two pneumococcal vaccines for healthy adults age 65 or older. They should get the Prevnar vaccine first and the Pneumovax vaccine one year later.

You also might need Tdap (tetanus, diphtheria, pertussis [whooping cough]) and hepatitis B vaccines.

38 Do you need a hepatitis B shot?

There's no one-size-fits-all answer to this question. Although most diabetes patients have compromised immune systems, you may still not need a hepatitis B shot.

Consider the following: Do you live in a hurricane/flooding area? Are you caring for infants and young children? The incontinent elderly? Are you planning to take a cruise or to travel to exotic places? If you answer "yes" to any of these questions, then my primary physician recommends a hepatitis B shot.

Otherwise you probably don't need one, although she suggests discussing whether you need the shot at every appointment, or when your plans change.

39 Take a multivitamin.

A daily multivitamin/mineral may reduce infections in people with type 2 diabetes. In a study reported in *Annals of Internal Medicine*, one group of type 2 diabetics took a daily multivitamin; the control group took a placebo (inert pill). After a year, only 17% of the vitamin group reported an infectious illness, compared with 93% who took the placebo. And the vitamin group reported *no* work-related absences, compared with 89% taking the placebo who reported at least one absence.

40 Enjoy your cup of joe.

Coffee reduces diabetes risk. Actually, it's the caffeine in coffee that makes it so beneficial. Since caffeine is often considered a drug, I've put this tip in the "drugs" chapter.

Harvard Public Health researchers followed 41,934 men form 1986 to 1998 and 84,276 women from 1980 to 1998. None of the study participants had diabetes at the beginning of the study. Men who drank more than six cups of caffeinated coffee per day cut their risk of type 2 diabetes by about 50%. Women who drank six cups cut their risk by 30%. The Harvard researchers theorized that caffeine affects the way the body metabolizes sugar, thus lowering the risk of type 2 diabetes.

Note: There was a more modest effect among decaf drinkers (25% risk reduction for men and 15% for women), and no statistically significant connection between type 2 diabetes and tea, although it also contains caffeine.

The study, published in the January 2004 issue of *Annals of Internal Medicine,* concluded that long-term coffee consumption is associated with a statistically significant lower risk of type 2 diabetes. So enjoy! Just stay away from those high-calorie, high-sugar coffee beverage blends that entice us at (almost) every street corner.

41 Congestive heart failure? Don't take these diabetes drugs.

The FDA has warned explicitly that *metformin* (Glucophage) and thiazolidenediones (TZDs) (such as Actos) should not be taken by diabetes patients with congestive heart failure.

Unfortunately, the use of these diabetes drugs has risen over the past decade. One study recently showed that a significant percentage of hospitalized Medicare recipients with both diseases were discharged with a *metformin* or TZD prescription.

If you suffer from both congestive heart failure and diabetes, ask your doctor to prescribe diabetes drugs that do not worsen congestive heart failure.

42 Is the pen mightier than the syringe?

Well, insulin pens—both prefilled disposable pens and insulin cartridges in reusable pens—are more convenient than syringes. And the pens are very accurate, especially for low doses of insulin.

One of the problems with greater U.S. adoption of insulin pens is that the FDA considers prefilled disposable pens to be drugs because they are self-contained. As such, they are often reimbursed by insurance companies. In contrast, reusable pens are generally not reimbursed, although the insulin cartridges are. Medicare does not cover syringes.

However, this is an area that is still evolving. In Europe, most insulin-dependent diabetics already use reusable insulin pens, which are covered by many countries' health systems.

43 Learn to lance without wincing.

Many insulin-dependent individuals with diabetes don't mind injecting insulin, but they hate checking their blood sugar. And the great majority of type 2 diabetics really hate the procedure because the lancing device is hard to use or it penetrates too deeply and painfully. It's definitely worth considering using lancets without the device and its scary, uncomfortable trigger. Or choose a device with a dial-a-depth feature, so that you can use different depth settings for different fingers.

44 Do the pill drill.

Get a pill container marked with the days of the week and seven to 21 compartments, depending on your needs. Fill it once a week, then use it every day.

This strategy has two advantages. First, you save time by doing this job once, rather than every day. Second, you know immediately whether you have taken your medications, rather than the occasional "Did I or didn't I?"

45 Testing your fingertips? Try this!

Before testing, soak your hand in hot water for several minutes. It will be much easier to get a sample when your blood rushes to the top of your skin.

46 Give your fingertips a rest.

Unless you are checking for hypoglycemia, when only your fingertips will give you an accurate result, use other sites to test your blood-glucose levels...and give your fingertips a rest.

Try your forearm, upper arm, calf, thigh, or the palm of your hand several inches below your thumb or your pinkie, close to your wrist. These areas have fewer nerve endings, so testing there will usually be less painful.

47 Take your pills properly.

Get the full benefit from your medications by understanding what the instructions mean.

"Before meals"—at least one hour before eating.

"After meals"—at least two hours after eating.

"With food"—during or just after a meal, not with just a glass of juice or milk.

"On an empty stomach"—one hour before or two hours after eating.

48 Beware of online pharmacies.

Ordering over the Internet can be tempting, and millions of people do. While many e-pharmacies are legitimate and require a faxed or mailed prescription from a licensed doctor who has examined you, many others are not. They will supply drugs without prescriptions. Sometimes people can get them by listing fake symptoms on the sites' medical questionnaires.

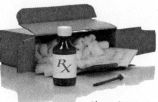

Photo: Spiritartist

Online drugs may not be such a bargain. Many e-pharmacies inflate their "bargain" prices with enormous consultation and shipping fees. And some sites can steal your money and personal identity.

To protect yourself, use only sites authorized by the Verified Internet Pharmacy Practice Sites program, identified on the online pharmacy's website. Make sure the sites are secure, so that your credit card information can't be stolen, and never give out your Social Security number or passwords.

The bottom line? Buyer beware.

49 Translate your glycosylated hemoglobin A1C numbers.

It may be difficult to relate the single-digit hemoglobin A1C percentages to two- and three-digit blood glucose figures. *Here's a sample table to show translations...*

A1C	ESTIMATED AVERAGE GLUCOSE
5%	97
6	126
7	154
8	183
9	212
10	240
11	269
12	298
13	326

Sources: Professional.Diabetes.org, DiabetesinControl.com

There are several A1C/blood glucose conversion calculators available online. The formula is (28.7 x A1C)– 46.7 = eAG.

That said, a difference of 0.2-0.5 between two tests is not serious and is not statistically significant. A difference of a whole percentage point is.

50 Know that your hemoglobin A1C number can be a moving target.

The hemoglobin A1C number of 7.0 or less—tight blood-glucose control— may be too aggressive as you get older. Excessively tight control can cause hypoglycemia, leading to dizziness, falls, and other problems.

Accordingly, the American Diabetes Association and the American Geriatrics Society advise an A1C goal of 7.5 if you have few medical issues and an A1C goal of 8.0 to 8.5 for patients who have multiple chronic illnesses and/or mild to moderate cognitive impairment, or are 65 years and older.

51 Realize that the glycosylated hemoglobin A1C number is an average.

Like the story of the man who drowned in a pond whose average depth was only 18 inches, it's possible to have a "good" reading of 6% (126 blood glucose) that is really an arithmetic average of much higher and lower numbers.

52 Don't reuse lancets.

Well, if you absolutely must, make sure that you've sterilized them by soaking them in rubbing alcohol. Reusing lancets to check your blood glucose raises the risk of dangerous finger infections. In rare cases, when lancets are used many times, these infections can become persistent and very difficult to cure.

53 Better blood-glucose control can lead to less medication.

Sometimes better control—achieving lower blood-sugar numbers—can mean reducing the dosage of your oral hypoglycemic drugs. Some of my friends have cut their *metformin* dosage in half, from 1,000 mg twice a day to one dose (1,000 mg) after breakfast.

And sometimes better control can mean cutting down on insulin or, in the case of people with type 2 diabetes, getting off insulin completely and using oral medication alone.

54 Don't get prescriptions filled on Sunday.

This may sound like the old slogan, "Don't buy a car built on Monday"—and it is.

Pharmacists who fill in on Sundays are usually not familiar with all the drugs that all their customers are taking. They don't know enough to question when something looks wrong, whether it's the prescription itself or just the insurance copayment. One Sunday I was charged the wrong price for a prescription—and didn't realize it until I got home because I was given a 30-day supply instead of the usual 90-day supply. That's how and why I wrote this tip.

55 Note the big difference between 70/30 insulin and 75/25 insulin.

It looks like just a 5% differential but it's a big difference that may make mealtimes easier for you.

Both are premixed insulins. However, the 70/30 mixture should be injected 30 to 45 minutes before eating. The 75/25 mixture, which contains fast-acting Humalog, is injected 15 minutes before eating, giving you greater flexibility.

56 Two separate insulins may work better for you.

Some insulin-dependent diabetics achieve better control from being able to calibrate specific doses of both their long- and short-acting insulins, rather than being locked into just increasing or decreasing the number of units of a fixed blend.

It can take several months for you and your doctor to figure out which system works better for you. Keeping a careful diary of blood-glucose readings, diet, and exercise is crucial.

57 Your insulin shouldn't be ice-cold.

If you keep your insulin in the refrigerator and injecting it hurts, take your vial(s) out before you inject so that the insulin will be at room temperature. That will make it less painful.

58 Rotate your injection sites.

You can always use the same, least painful area of your body so long as you rotate your injection sites. For example, you can always inject insulin into your abdomen—avoiding the area around your navel—if you rotate the exact location.

One easy method is to picture your abdomen as a clock and place each injection at the next hour marking. When you have circled the clock on the left side of your belly, switch to the right. That will give you plenty of time to heal and avoid internal scarring, which can affect the proper absorption of the insulin.

59 Some insulins can be injected anywhere, some can't.

Slower-acting insulins like Lantus and the new drugs covered at the end of this chapter can be injected anywhere in the body where there is enough fat to avoid injecting into muscle tissue. (Ask your doctor if unsure.) But Humalog and other new fast-acting insulins should be injected only into the abdomen so that it is absorbed most rapidly.

60 Check your prescriptions before you leave the pharmacy.

Go one step further than just checking the label. Open the bottle and examine the pills themselves. If a pill looks different from what you're used to, check that the code printed on the pill is identical to the code printed on the label.

(The website RxList.com lets you type in the code and get the name and the dosage of the drug, or ask the pharmacist to do it for you.)

Note: Sometimes a pharmacy may substitute twice as many pills that are half your usual dosage if it runs out of your prescribed dose, but your pharmacist should instruct you to take twice as many of the pills.

61 Use a national pharmacy chain.

You're in a faraway city when suddenly you realize that you forgot to pack your medications. That's no problem if you use a national pharmacy chain. Just ask the pharmacist in the city you're visiting to check your prescription online, explain that you need a week's refill of your medications, and you'll be able to get them quickly and easily.

62 Get familiar with the formulary.

Most health-insurance plans have a formulary—a list of brand-name and generic drugs for which they will pay, and leave you with the usually reasonable copay.

But if your doctor prescribes a drug that is not in the formulary, you will have to pay the full retail price, and it can be horrendous. For example, Cipro antibiotic ear drops, which were not in my medical group's formulary, cost $110; Cortisporin, a similar brand-name antibiotic ear drop, cost only $18 at Walmart.

To save yourself time and aggravation, when your doctor gives you a new prescription, ask whether the drug is in the formulary. If your doctor doesn't know, ask whether the prescription can be written so that an equivalent formulary-acceptable brand-name or generic drug can be substituted.

63 Moving to insulin doesn't mean you've failed.

Over time, many people with type 2 diabetes will progress from taking oral medications to needing to take insulin. This does not signify failure. It simply means that your pancreas is producing less insulin, so supplementing your body's own supply of insulin is now necessary. Your doctor can refer you to a diabetes educator who will teach you how to inject and store insulin. (It's really easy!)

64 Beat insulin weight gain.

Many people with type 2 diabetes who are put on insulin for better blood-glucose control discover that their weight skyrockets 20 to 50 pounds within the first year. *If this has been your experience, here's why it happened, and here's how to solve the problem…*

Before you started on insulin, your body was not able to metabolize carbohydrates efficiently, so the glucose that was produced was excreted in your urine, rather than going into your cells to be used. But on insulin, your body is able to use all those carbohydrates, hence the weight gain.

With all those calories and carbohydrates being used now, you won't feel as hungry or eat as much, but it will take time for your body to adjust...and you may actually gain weight. Of course you should be working on weight control through diet and exercise, but if you start packing on "insulin pounds," talk to your doctor. Your dosage may need to be increased. (This may sound perplexing at first, but remember, increased insulin makes you *less* hungry.)

65 Know that vitamin E may reduce the risk of type 2 diabetes.

A long-term Finnish study (1967-1995) reported in the February 27, 2004, issue of *Diabetes Care* concluded that there was a significant correlation between diets higher in vitamin E and a reduced risk of type 2 diabetes.

Vitamin E is also essential for cardiovascular health. It acts as a blood thinner, which reduces the risk of clots and helps keep LDL (bad) cholesterol from forming plaques that stick to artery walls and may cause blockages.

Curiously, there was no statistical correlation between vitamin C and reduced risk of type 2 diabetes.

Note: While vitamin E is technically a supplement, I've included it in the "drugs" chapter because it's being used in a drug-like manner.

66 Know that diuretics can raise your blood glucose.

This tip may sound like the computer error message: "It's not my fault …" But if you have just been put on a diuretic (water pill) to lower your blood pressure, the concentration of glucose in your blood will probably rise.

If your high blood glucose lasts more than two or three days while your body gets used to the diuretic, call your doctor. You may need to increase your insulin or hypoglycemic-drug dosage, or use a lower dosage of the diuretic, or a different one.

67 Know your *metformin* drug interactions.

Metformin and other hypoglycemic drugs are excellent and safe for many patients.

But, according to Drugs.com, metformin can interact with 683 drugs: 14 major, 610 moderate, and 59 minor reactions.

Check with your doctor and pharmacist to see whether metformin interacts with any of your other drugs, and if changes may be necessary.

68 Get your pharmacy's package insert.

This long strip of paper with its tiny print and biochemical vocabulary is definitely worth reading, even if you have to research the definitions of many technical terms. Fortunately, the most important information is printed in bold type in clear English, e.g., "WARNINGS: Diabetes and Hypoglycemia…"

69 Keep a small supply of pain pills handy.

This tip is not for everyone, but it really works. It depends on your having a good, long-running relationship with your doctor, who knows that you are a conscientious patient and do not have an addictive personality.

People with diabetes often have episodes of pain—especially in the winter. Having a 10-day supply of pain pills can alleviate pain which in turn, will lower their blood-glucose levels.

Besides pill splitting (Tip 27) and asking your doctor to prescribe generic drugs, here are other ways to pay less for your medications…

70 Pay less for prescription drugs I: Ask your doctor for samples.

Doctors always have sample drugs to give out to their patients. But if you don't say, "Do you have any samples of this?" you won't get any freebies. Your simple request can save you big bucks—especially if the drug is being prescribed for the first time and you don't know how you'll react. But it's also a good idea to ask for samples even if you've been taking the drug for a while.

71 Pay less for prescription drugs II: How to save if there's no generic.

Some drugs are still covered by patent, so no generics are available. To find out if there is a generic equivalent, check the *FDA's Electronic Orange Book* (officially titled *Approved Drug Products With Therapeutic Equivalence Evaluations*) online at the FDA website, FDA.gov.

If your prescription is not available as a generic, ask your doctor if there is a *similar*, less expensive drug that can be prescribed instead.

72 Pay less for prescription drugs III: Buy through mail order.

The mail-order pharmacies discussed here are completely different from the online pharmacies I warned you about earlier in this chapter (Tip 48). These mail-order pharmacies have real addresses and phone numbers, and some of them are divisions of companies listed on the stock exchanges.

One simple way to find a reliable mail-order pharmacy is to ask your doctor or someone you trust for recommendations. Another is to look carefully at the pharmacy's website to check whether it requires a prescription from your doctor and whether it displays the logo that it is a secure website prominently.

These mail-order pharmacies can save their customers money because they may be located in low-rent or low-tax areas. Comparison-shop carefully. These mail-order pharmacies may be worth using just because they are so convenient; most guarantee delivery in less than five days.

Before you order, ask the pharmacy how it will deal with replacing your prescription if you forget it when you travel.

73 Pay less for prescription drugs IV: Buy your drugs in bulk.

This strategy works especially well if you are taking prescription drugs for chronic or long-term problems. Unless doctors think you might misuse a drug, they are usually willing to write prescriptions for larger quantities, and pharmacies will fill those economy-sized prescriptions—unless they are limited by insurance companies.

How much can you save? One national pharmacy chain charges $11-$13 for a one-month supply (thirty 20 mg pills) of *atorvastatin*, a commonly prescribed generic hypertension drug. But a three-month supply of the same drug cost only about $20 with a downloadable coupon. The savings were amazing!

74 Pay less for prescription drugs V: Ask for a substitute.

Even if your doctor hasn't indicated that a generic drug can be substituted, ask your pharmacist about making the substitution. In most states, unless a prescription is marked specifically "Dispense as written," pharmacists are permitted to substitute the generic version of the proprietary (brand-name) drug.

75 Pay less for prescription drugs VI: The key question to ask.

Many people with diabetes will be taking the same prescription drugs for the rest of their lives. Nevertheless, as advised in Tip 33, always ask your doctor, especially on repeat visits or when you are getting refill prescriptions, "Is it still necessary for me to take this drug?" It may not be—or something newer and better may have come along since your last visit.

76 Pay less for prescription drugs VII: Fill them in December.

If you spend lots of money on drugs, as many of us diabetics do, you will have passed Medicare's "hole in the doughnut" sometime in the fall. As a result, if you get your prescriptions filled in December, your copays can be more than *90% lower*. For example, my prescription for *lidocaine* pain patches, which cost me a $70 copayment in the spring of 2016, cost me only $2.95 in December!

Such savings can also happen if you have a high-deductible health insurance plan...once you meet the deductible.

Along with knowing how to save on your drugs, it's important to know what's "new and approved"...

77 Recent drugs I: "Newer" may not be "better."

We're all tempted to believe that newer drugs MUST be better; otherwise, why were they developed? But because they ARE new, they just don't have the history of risks and side effects of older drugs. This is especially important if you have kidney disease.

How to finesse this problem? Ask your endocrinologist and your nephrologist about the risks and side effects of any newly prescribed diabetes drugs and monitor them for at least one month. Are they lowering your blood glucose? Are you having any side effects?

78 Recent drugs II: Take advantage of those glorious coupons.

Any time your doctor puts you on a new drug, see if there's a downloadable coupon for it on the drug's website. With these coupons, it's possible to pay only $5-$25 per prescription if you qualify—and most of us do!

79 Recent drugs III: Afrezza.

Afrezza is an inhalable insulin. In June 2014 the FDA approved Afrezza for both types 1 and 2 diabetics, with a label restriction for patients having asthma, active lung cancer, or chronic obstruction pulmonary disease (COPD). It is a rapid-acting insulin, so patients must also use a long-acting insulin.

80 Recent drugs IV: Basaglar.

Basaglar, which has the same amino-acid sequences as Lantus, is the first insulin to be approved through an abbreviated process and is delivered via the Basaglar KwikPen, a prefilled pen containing 300 units of the drug.

81 Recent drugs V: Farxiga.

Farxiga, an oral drug for type 2 diabetes, was approved by the FDA in January 2014. It is taken in the morning in a 5 mg or 10 mg dose. Taking Farxiga leads to heavy excretion of sugar in the urine, lowering blood glucose, but also causing rapid weight loss, fatigue, and dehydration. If you are taking Farxiga, make sure to keep up your fluid intake.

82 Recent drugs VI: Invokana.

Invokana was approved by the FDA in March 2013 and became the first drug of its type in the United States.

This once-daily oral medication for type 2 diabetes is taken in doses of 100 mg to 300 mg. The higher dose has been proved to show greater hemoglobin A1C reductions than Januvia, with the majority of patients reaching an A1C goal of less than 7%.

However, Invokana possesses side effects—increased incidence of urinary-tract infections, elevations in LDL (bad) cholesterol, increased urination, episodes of low blood pressure, and possibly the risk of diabetic ketoacidosis, described fully in Tip 1055, and possible cardiovascular problems.

83 Recent drugs VII: Jardiance.

Jardiance is an oral hypoglycemic drug used to lower blood glucose in patients with type 2 diabetes. Approved by the FDA in August 2014, it is taken once a day, in the morning. In a clinical trial published in the *New England Journal of Medicine* and reported in the *New York Times* on September 17, 2015, Jardiance was shown to reduce deaths from cardiovascular disease by 38%, mostly from heart failure.

Jardiance is not recommended for patients who have kidney disease or who are on dialysis, or who have diabetic ketoacidosis.

84 Recent drugs VIII: Levemir.

Levemir is a long-acting injectable insulin for type 1 and type 2 diabetics who need better control of their blood glucose and hemoglobin A1C, available since 2014. Levemir comes in a prefilled insulin pen (Levemir FlexTouch), which contains 300 units. Once the package is unsealed, Levemir can last 42 days without refrigeration.

85 Recent drugs IX: LixiLan.

LixiLan is a combination of the familiar long-acting Lantus and Lyxumia, a once-daily injectable drug for poorly controlled type 2 diabetes. It received FDA approval in 2016. Discuss with your doctor if this drug is right for you.

86 Recent drugs X: Ryzodeg.

Available since 2015, Ryzodeg contains a combination of short- and long-acting insulin in a pen. The drug starts to work within 10 to 20 minutes, peaks in about one hour, and keeps on working for 24 hours or longer. It is used for type 1 and type 2 diabetes patients.

Because Ryzodeg is premixed, your doctor will have to monitor your blood glucose carefully until the correct dosage can be determined.

87 Recent drugs XI: Toujeo.

Toujeo is a new basal insulin in a pen which has a higher concentration of insulin than the long-established Lantus (U-300 instead of the familiar U-100), meaning that patients can inject fewer units. It was approved by the FDA in February 2015. It is prescribed for type 2 diabetes.

However, many patients reported dissatisfaction and gave the drug low ratings because they found it ineffective and had to keep increasing their dosage.

88 Recent drugs XII: Tresiba.

Tresiba is a new basal insulin in a pen that has double the concentration of Lantus (U-200 vs. the familiar U-100). It comes in a 160-unit pen.

Approved by the FDA in December 2016, the manufacturer claims that the drug is very predictable and stable. It has a half-life of 25 hours and can last at least 42 hours. As such, it would be useful for diabetic patients with uneven insulin and meal schedules.

89 Recent drugs XIII: Trulicity.

Approved by the FDA in September 2014, Trulicity is a once-weekly injection that normalizes blood-glucose levels in type 2 diabetics. It is designed to work alone or in combination with such other drugs as *metformin*, sulfonylureas, and insulin, all taken with meals.

90 Recent drugs XIV: Victoza.

Victoza is a once-daily injectable drug approved by the FDA for type 2 diabetes in 2010 and a variant dose (Saxenda) in 2015 for adults with a Body Mass Index (BMI) of 30 or greater (obese) or a BMI of 27 or greater (overweight) who have at least one weight-related condition.

Some serious side effects have been reported—pancreatitis, pancreatic cancer, and thyroid tumors—but the jury is still out on a *demonstrated* causal connection.

91 Recent drugs XV: Xultophy.

Xultophy is a combination of the fairly new Tresiba and Victoza (see Tips 88 and 90), designed for once-daily injection for type 2 diabetes. It was approved by the FDA in November 2016. Ask your diabetes doctor whether Xultophy might help you.

92 Lab-grown insulin may be on the way.

In April 2016 the Gene Expression Laboratory at the Salk Institute for Biological Studies reported that its scientists had discovered a master genetic switch key for prompting pancreatic beta cells, which normally detect and respond to sugar in the blood, to grow patient-derived functioning beta cells for transplant in a potential new diabetes therapy.

93 Implantable insulin delivery pump.

Intarcia Therapeutics, a privately held Hayward, California, company, has cleared its FDA Phase III trials in its Medici Drug Delivery System, an implantable diabetes-drug-delivery pump. The 2" matchstick-sized rods are designed to last six to 12 months, implanted in the abdomen just beneath the skin by a physician or physician's assistant. The procedure should take five minutes.

CHAPTER 2

Weight Loss and Nutrition

AUTHOR'S NOTE
No Diet Is Right for Everyone

As long-term dieters know, there is no "one-size-fits-all" diet. What works for you may not work for me, and vice versa. Although we both have diabetes, our body chemistry may be different, with one of us being able to metabolize carbohydrates fairly easily, with the help of oral hypoglycemics or insulin, and the other having trouble metabolizing those same carbohydrates, despite the help of oral hypoglycemics or insulin.

It may sound simplistic to say, "Do what works for you," but most of us have lived long enough to know whether we flourish under a high-carbohydrate or low-carbohydrate diet. Which diet helps us lose weight? Which one gives us more energy? Which one gives us better blood-glucose readings?

Many of the tips in this chapter have a low-carbohydrate bias because their contributors benefited from a low-carbohydrate diet and, probably, because they were disgruntled about being told constantly to go on a high-carbohydrate diet when empirically it made no sense to them. They had not succeeded with high-carbohydrate diets.

If I had to choose, I would stay away from the extremes of high- and low-carbohydrate diets. Probably neither 300 grams nor 30 grams of carbohydrate a day is healthful. A middle ground seems more sensible to me, more "Mediterranean" than Atkins Induction. Of course, the carbohydrates we choose should be complex, rather than simple and digested too quickly.

But that's just my humble opinion, and what's worked for me. Whatever diet you choose, have it checked by your doctor or Certified Diabetes Educator.

94 Sugar in cigarettes? *Surprise!!!*

There's lots of sugar in cigarette tobacco—so much so that I've made this Tip #1 in this chapter. Unfortunately, cigarette manufacturers don't have to list sugar content on the package the way they do nicotine and tar.

Would it surprise you to learn that cigarette tobacco contains approximately 20% sugar? Would it help you quit smoking and lose weight?

(I was a three-pack-a-day smoker, but quit cold turkey in 1963. I chewed up lots of pencils and knitted lots of scarves in that first year without cigarettes.)

95 Stay away from your "trigger" foods.

We all have a love-hate relationship with certain foods: The ones that sing their siren song to us until we open the package—and then consume its entire contents. And then we feel guilty as all get-out.

Very often, measuring out small portions of these beloved trigger foods doesn't work. We go back again and again and again.

The only effective strategy is to stay away from those foods completely—or to find a safer substitute, like air-popped popcorn instead of potato chips.

96 Better than breading.

Most ingredients used to bread meat or fish for sauteing contain large percentages of carbohydrates: white or whole-wheat flour, even nutritious wheat germ.

Finely chopped almonds are a better breading choice. The nuts contain protein, minerals, a little fat, and only a trace of carbohydrate. And they add lots of flavor and texture to your recipe.

Big carb savings: One-quarter cup of all-purpose flour contains 24 grams of carbohydrate; one-quarter cup of chopped almonds only 6 grams.

97 Create beauty with origami.

I've put this tip into the "Weight Loss and Nutrition" chapter for a sneaky reason: Making origami prevents you from snacking for hours at a time.

Folding those beautiful papers so intricately and following complex instructions requires concentration. It's impractical to stop in the middle to grab a cookie, chip, or pretzel, then have to wash your hands and try to find your place again before continuing to create your origami pretties.

98 Start with soup.

Hot or cold, soup makes an excellent starter. As you sip or spoon it, your brain and stomach begin to feel full. Consequently, you are likely to eat less of your main course and will consume fewer total calories. In fact, many successful diet plans are based on soup.

Here are some suggestions for quick, easy soups…

COLD: For all of these, you will need a blender and one to two cups of lowfat buttermilk per portion. Put the buttermilk in the blender. For Scandinavian-style fruit soups—so delicious in hot weather!—add one-half to one cup of cut-up fresh apricots, cherries, raspberries, strawberries, or blueberries. As an extra treat, add one teaspoon rum, cognac, amaretto, or almond extract. Blend, chill, and serve.

For cream of spinach, start with one to two cups of lowfat buttermilk per portion and put in blender. Thaw one-half of a 10-ounce package of frozen chopped spinach, press out the water, and place in blender. Blend, chill, and serve. Marvelous with grated nutmeg sprinkled on top.

HOT: Choose a low-sodium beef or chicken broth. Some bouillon cubes are excellent. Boil with chopped vegetables—celery, carrots, spinach, onions, etc.—until veggies are tender. Top with fresh or freeze-dried parsley.

99 Soup can make a meal.

Take all the benefits in the preceding tip—and multiply them.

When you make soup your dinner, you are filling up on lots of low-calorie fluid. *Here are two quick dinners based on revved-up soups…*

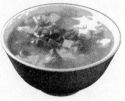

Exotic egg-drop: Heat a can of chicken broth. Add a well-drained can of chicken breast and/or two beaten eggs, swirled with a fork through the soup. This is "egg drop" (without the high-carb cornstarch of the Cantonese version) or what Italian cooks call *stracciatella*. Top with fresh or dried chives.

Photo: whitewish

Easy, elegant crabmeat soup: Saute some chopped onion in unsalted butter, add one and one-half cup of lowfat buttermilk (or regular lowfat milk) and a well-drained six-ounce can of crabmeat. Add a quarter teaspoon of curry powder or for an extra treat, add one teaspoon cognac or dry sherry…the alcohol and calories will evaporate. Heat thoroughly and serve.

100 Guilt-free potato chips.

When you have an overpowering urge for potato chips, make your own to cut calories, carbohydrates, and fat. Store-bought chips are high in all three, so those snacks can really wreck your diet. For example, one company's potato chips contain 150 calories, 10 grams of fat, and 25 grams of carbohydrates in a one-ounce serving. The company's baked variety contains 110 calories and only 1.5 grams of fat, but still has 23 grams of carbohydrate in a one-ounce serving.

This recipe has only one disadvantage: You have to start the simple preparation the night before or the morning of your splurge.

Fill a two- or three-quart bowl with cold water. Scrub one or two potatoes; leave them unpeeled for extra minerals and flavor. Cut into thin slices, put into bowl of water, and refrigerate for at least eight hours. Then remove the potato slices with a slotted spoon or spatula and place on a paper towel to dry.

You will notice that the bowl of water has a lot of white powder at the bottom. This is potato starch, which has been leached out of the potato slices, and is the source of most of the calories and carbohydrates.

Preheat your oven to 400 degrees. Spray a cookie sheet with vegetable spray—use butter or olive-oil flavor for extra taste. Place the potato slices on the cookie sheet in a single layer. Bake eight to 10 minutes per side until golden brown. Serve.

I'd love to be able to give you a calorie and carbohydrate count for this recipe, but there are too many variables. The thinner you slice the potatoes and the longer they sit in the ice water, the more starch will be removed, and the lower the calorie and carbohydrate count will be. (The calories and fat grams in the cooking spray are negligible.) My estimate is that this recipe has only 30 to 40 calories and five grams of carbohydrate per one-ounce serving.

101 The joys of Jell-O. Sugar-free, that is.

It's a perfect bingeing food because an entire package (four ½-cup servings) contains only 40 calories and 0 grams of carbohydrate. In contrast, one ½-cup serving of the sugary variety contains 80 calories and 19 grams of carbohydrate. The whole bowl (ouch!): 320 calories and 76 grams of carbohydrate.

Back to the sugar-free…jazz it up by combining two flavors: lemon and lime, raspberry and strawberry, cherry and cranberry. Substitute plain or flavored seltzer for the cold water. Or add small pieces of fresh or sugar-free frozen fruit or berries. For a patriotic, colorful dessert, prepare one of the red flavors and refrigerate about 1½ hours, or until thickened. Stir in fresh blueberries and refrigerate 4 hours, or until firm.

102 Have a guiltless BLT.

Pan-broil three strips of turkey bacon. Layer with a sliced tomato on a leaf of romaine. Wrap and eat.

Approximately 90 calories, 6 grams of carbohydrate, 9 grams of protein, and only 1.5 grams of fat.

103 Chocolate fix I: Chocolate milk.

Making your own chocolate syrup is a calorie and carbohydrate bargain. One brand's two-tablespoon serving of chocolate syrup has 100 calories and 25 grams of carbohydrate, 20 of them sugar. Another brand has 120 calories and 29 grams of carbohydrate, 23 of them sugar. Even a "lite" version has 50 calories and 12 grams of carbohydrate, 10 of them sugar.

My own chocolate syrup has 40 calories per two-tablespoon serving, but only six grams of carbohydrate—no sugar. It also packs two grams of fiber into each serving. Put two tablespoons of plain (baking) cocoa into a large glass. Add three envelopes of Equal or a similar sweetener and two to three tablespoons of hot water. Stir well to make a syrup, add low-fat or skim milk, and stir again. Drink up guiltlessly!

You can also rev up this syrup with almond, rum, or brandy flavoring. Try it in your coffee for a very low-calorie treat.

104 Check food labels before you buy.

Little differences in calories, carbohydrates, and fat between brands add up.

One brand of garlic and herb pasta sauce has 110 calories per ½-cup serving, with 17 grams of carbohydrate including 11 grams of sugar, 4 grams of fat, and 2 grams each of fiber and protein.

A "healthier" competitor has only 50 calories per ½-cup serving, with 11 grams of carbohydrate including eight grams of sugar, 0 grams of fat, and 3 grams each of fiber and protein—less than half the calories, two-thirds of the carbohydrates, and more fiber and protein.

105 Chocolate fix II: Rum or cognac truffles.

I created this recipe for my chocoholic diabetic and nondiabetic friends. The truffles' flavor is so incredibly intense that just one or two are luxuriously satisfying. And each truffle contains only 3 grams of carbohydrate.

1 7 oz. bar Hershey's Special Dark Chocolate

5 oz. unsweetened baking chocolate

7 Tbsp. heavy cream

3 Tbsp. dark rum or cognac

½ cup (approximately) raw or blanched almonds, chopped fine

Break the chocolate into small pieces and place in large heatproof bowl.

In a heavy saucepan, bring the cream to just boiling and pour over the chocolate. Let sit for five minutes and stir until smooth.

Add rum or cognac and stir again.

Cover bowl and refrigerate three hours to overnight.

With a melon baller, scoop and shape truffles, then roll them in chopped almonds.

Keep in a covered container. Serve at room temperature.

Yield: Approximately 50 truffles; 60 calories and 3 grams of carbohydrate per truffle.

Variation: Substitute Grand Marnier or Sabra liqueur for the rum or cognac, and add grated orange zest to the chopped almonds for rolling the truffles. Approximately 70 calories and 4 grams of carbohydrate per truffle.

106 Magic in mushrooms.

I can't think of many foods that are as delicious and as low-calorie, low-carbohydrate, and low-fat as mushrooms. Most varieties of mushrooms contain less than 30 calories, 2 grams of carbohydrate, and only a trace of fat in a ½-cup portion.

Some mushrooms possess valuable medicinal properties, too. The Chinese mushroom known as the black tree ear has proved to be an anticoagulant, similar to aspirin. It may help prevent narrowed arteries—a cause of high blood pressure—and clots that are a special concern for us diabetics.

Shiitake mushrooms contain lentinan, a strong antiviral substance that kills many viruses, stimulates the immune system, and lowers cholesterol when eaten daily.

Recent research out of Tufts Medical School and the USDA Human Nutrition Research Center, published in the May 8, 2014, issue of the *Journal of Nutrition,* suggests that various species of mushrooms can help in weight reduction as a meat extender that does not sacrifice flavor.

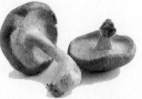
Photo: Elenathewise

107 Mock not the cucumber.

Cucumbers are an energy booster. Many people with diabetes find that cucumbers are low in carbohydrates, but high in B vitamins, fiber, and liquid. A cuke break can give you a healthier energy boost, without the after-crash of coffee or canned or bottled energy drinks.

108 Quick gazpacho.

Mix one-half cup of "healthy" (no sugar) garlic and herb pasta sauce with one-half cup of water. Chill. Top with diced red, yellow, and green pepper and/or chives and parsley.

Approximately 50 calories, 11 grams carbohydrate, 3 grams protein, 0 grams fat.

109 Be wary of "diabetic" cookbooks.

A helpful friend recently gave me a cookbook that had "sugar-free" right in its title. However, a careful reading of the cover "explained" that the recipes used only "all-natural sweeteners."

What does this mean? Honey, date sugar, apple-juice concentrate, dried figs, brown-rice syrup, raisins—often more than one in the same recipe.

The per-serving data reveal that most people with diabetes and dieters would shun this book. Most of the recipes contain 200 calories and 30 grams of carbohydrate per serving; one recipe for Apple Spice Cake contained 295 calories and 38 grams of carbohydrate per slice. That's roughly 20% of my daily calories and 30% of my daily carbohydrates. Of the more than 100 recipes in this cookbook, I found only a scant handful that met my calorie and carbohydrate requirements, so I gave the cookbook to the library.

110 Let yourself splurge once a week.

One of the most successful dieters I know has kept his weight loss for over 20 years. His secret? He watches his calories, carbohydrates, and fats six days a week, but on Saturday or Sunday, he lets himself feast a little. The next day, he's back to watching his food intake.

111 Cut the fat, cut the calories I.

Trim all fat off meat before broiling, roasting, or stewing it.

112 Cut the fat, cut the calories II.

Broil or roast meat in a ridged aluminum foil pan. The meat will sit and cook on the ridges while the fat drains below, away from the meat.

113 Cut the fat, cut the calories III.

Blot broiled or roasted meat with a paper towel or napkin before serving it. See how much fat is absorbed? This little trick also works beautifully on your monthly slice of pizza.

114 Choose chopsticks to slow down.

Use chopsticks for all kinds of food—not just Asian cuisine. You'll benefit greatly from using them at home. Chopsticks slow down your eating speed, so you'll feel full faster on less food. And slowing down will give you the opportunity to taste and enjoy your food more.

Chopsticks also let you exercise your fingers and hands without realizing it, which can reduce the risk of carpal tunnel syndrome and arthritis.

As an added bonus, learning to master chopsticks will make you smile at yourself and at the world.

115 Learn a new recipe every week.

Diet and nutrition are a full-time "job" for everyone concerned with optimum health. You'll get more joy out of that job by turning it into a pleasurable hobby.

Find and tweak unusual recipes for chicken, fish, dairy, grains, and fruits and vegetables. Will they taste better with more or different herbs or spices? Sure, you'll have some results that you wouldn't repeat, but so do professional chefs. At the end of a year, you should have at least 20 healthy new recipes to feast on.

116 Turn an appetizer into dinner.

This trick works especially well in hot weather, when you don't want to cook.

Supersize a shrimp or crabmeat cocktail for your main course. Start with six to eight ounces of chilled boiled shrimp or a can of crabmeat on a bed of lettuce or greens and top with two tablespoons of cocktail sauce (the sauce has approximately 10 calories, 3 grams of carbohydrate). Add a slice of whole-grain bread, if you like. Finish your feast with fresh fruit or berries.

A cheese plate with fruit and whole-grain crackers is another excellent choice.

117 Downsize your plate size.

Because you "eat with your eyes," a portion of food looks bigger if it's put on a smaller plate.

Take advantage of this strategy by substituting a salad plate for your dinner plate. The average salad plate is 60% the size of the average dinner plate—47 square inches vs. 79 square inches—so you'll cut back on your food intake without really being conscious that you're doing it.

And no going back for seconds, except for salad or green and yellow veggies.

118 Open-face your sandwiches.

When you make your sandwich with one slice of bread instead of two, you save approximately 80 calories and—even more important—16 grams of carbohydrate.

Unless you are brown-bagging your sandwich, it's better to make and eat an open sandwich because it has the same surface area as the usual two-slice variety. However, if you are packing your sandwich, cut the slice of bread in half, make a thick half-sandwich, and eat it very slowly.

119 Make chocolate part of your meal plan.

Chocolate lovers, rejoice! If you can stop at one or two squares of chocolate this tip is for you.

You probably already know the medical benefits of chocolate. It contains theobromine, a proven antidepressant, and resveratrol, the phytochemical in red wine that has been linked to a reduced risk of coronary disease and cancer.

Chocolate and a glass of 1% milk can be a nutritious occasional lunch. Forty grams (1½ ounces) of 85% dark chocolate "cost" 230 calories, with only 15 grams of carbohydrate, 6 grams of fiber (9 grams of net carbs) with 5 grams each of sugar and protein. Forty grams of 90% dark chocolate is an even better bet, "costing" 240 calories, but with only 12 grams of carbohydrate, 5 grams of fiber (7 grams of net carbs), *with only 3 grams of sugar* and 5 grams of protein. The milk adds 100 calories, 12 grams of carbohydrate, 8 grams of protein, and only 2.5 grams of fat. Your total will be 330 to 340 calories, with only 12 to 15 grams of carbohydrate, 7 to 9 grams of net carbs, 3 to 5 grams of sugar, and 5 grams of protein.

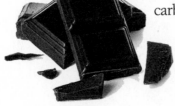

And—if you can find it—40 grams of 99% dark chocolate "cost" only 216 calories, with only 3 grams of carbohydrate, 2 grams of fiber (1 gram of net carbs), with less than 1 gram of sugar and over 5 grams of protein.

Photo: yvdavyd

This is *not* the kind of quickie meal to eat every day, but it provides enough nutritional and medical benefits to indulge in once or twice a week without feeling guilty.

120 Know the difference between hunger and thirst.

It sounds very simple, but in fact many people reach for food when they are really thirsty.

Check this for yourself by drinking a glass of ice water when you think you are hungry. Wait five minutes. Do you feel less hungry now? If not, have a little snack.

121 Being a gourmet won't wreck your budget.

You can feast on very little money. Take the time to shop for the freshest food; it may mean going to three or four stores instead of one mega supermarket.

Pass up junk food, fast food, and prepared food. They are usually too high in calories, fat, carbohydrates, and sodium.

Instead, do your food shopping European-style. Spend time choosing perfect meat, fish, and produce. They will be fresher than at the supermarkets, which use regional distribution. Take advantage of seasonal bargains. Once in a while, splurge on the exotic, like raspberries in the winter or doughnut peaches. Turn your butcher and produce manager into friends by asking their advice. Buy your whole-grain bread at the bakery on the morning they make it. Buy your rolls one at a time.

Aren't you worth all this extra work?

122 Plan your meals in advance...

It's easier to eat right if you plan your meals in advance. Read store flyers to learn about weekly specials, make shopping lists, and try to shop only once or twice a week. It's much smarter to buy "family packs" of meat at bargain prices, and then wrap and freeze single portions.

Many busy people cook in batches on weekends and freeze individual-sized portions, then just reheat and add a different salad or vegetable and dessert every night.

123 ...But give yourself some leeway.

Give yourself permission to be spontaneous, too. You may see some interesting food on display, or taste it in an in-store promotion, or even see it in another customer's grocery cart.

Be flexible: If it intrigues you, buy it and try it.

124 Jazz up your water.

Drinking those eight glasses of water day after day can become boring.

Change the taste by adding these flavorings...

- **Spearmint or peppermint extract**
- **One or two tablespoons of orange, apple, or pineapple juice**
- **Almond extract.** You can make a zero-calorie orzata (Italian almond syrup) with almond extract and Equal. Fill your glass with cold water.

Let these suggestions inspire you to experiment further!

125 Experiment with herbs and spices.

Herbs and spices can completely change the taste of bland foods and enhance the flavor of others.

You are familiar with black and red pepper, but there are dozens of varieties. There are even subtle differences among different types of sea salt.

Experiment with the more unusual herbs, both fresh and dried. You may use six or eight frequently, but there are at least two or three dozen in many supermarkets. You'll get maximum flavor from buying whole spices like mustard, allspice, cloves, nutmeg, and pepper, and grinding them yourself as you need them. (Doing this will also perfume your home.)

Although you should avoid prepared herbs containing salt (buy minced or powdered onion or garlic instead of onion or garlic salt), there are many other interesting combinations. Mrs. Dash makes over a dozen varieties—all salt-free.

126 Ditch the "I was good/I was bad" mind-set.

When you say to yourself or tell your friends, "I was good; I had fish and a salad for dinner yesterday." Or "I was bad; I had doughnuts for breakfast this morning," you are reverting to an emotional childhood, in which you are a good or bad kid out to either please or disobey Mommy or the latest authority figure—doctor, nutritionist, diabetes educator.

You have the power—not the authority figures, and certainly not the food. Instead of "good" or "bad," take the approach that if you overate at your last meal, you can eat less at the next one, and it will balance by the end of the day or the week. Every meal gives you a new opportunity to eat sensibly and healthfully.

127 Cancel your membership in the clean-plate club.

Our mothers may have taught us too well. They forced us to join the Clean Plate Club because children in Europe or Asia or Africa were starving, so we shouldn't waste our food. That was a sin, and they made us feel horribly guilty if we didn't eat every morsel.

Rise above that ancient guilt trip. You're an intelligent, independent adult now. It's better to waste money on food that you throw away than to spend it on doctors and drugs.

128 Take the glycemic index with a grain of salt.

The glycemic index is really an *average* obtained from the test results of many people. It is not a precise mathematical number.

"Average" means that some people with diabetes will react to a food with a high blood-glucose number, some with a low blood-glucose number, and most will fall somewhere in the middle. And many of those people will have significantly different blood-glucose numbers when they eat that food the next time, and the next.

Accordingly, many people with diabetes should pay more attention to the way individual high-carbohydrate foods affect *them*, as though they were having allergic reactions to those foods. For example, one of my type 1 friends can eat a potato or one half-cup of rice, and his evening blood glucose will rise only 20 to 30 points, where another type 1 friend's evening blood glucose will rise 70 to 80 points and will still be high the next morning.

129 Balance your nutrition by the week.

You don't have to balance every single meal nutritionally. It may be more convenient to achieve balance over an entire week or longer. Especially if you live alone, you may find it easier to eat the same lunch or dinner two or three days in a row. When shrimp is on sale, you may enjoy eating shrimp marinara several days in a row, followed by grilled shrimp brochettes, followed by shrimp stir-fry or shrimp salad.

Next week chicken, beef, or dairy may be on sale, and they will offer a basket of other nutritional benefits. Over a month, it all adds up and balances out.

130 Let your blood-glucose decide what and how much you will eat.

Many successful people with diabetes base their meal plans on their blood-glucose readings. For example, if their blood-glucose reading is 70-100, they may have a larger portion of carbohydrates…if it is 120-140, they may have an average portion…and if it is over 200, they may have a much smaller portion.

131 Enjoy festive foods—but in small portions.

Our lives would be very dreary without the foods we eat to celebrate birthdays, weddings, sweet sixteens, bar and bat mitzvahs, confirmations, graduations, Thanksgiving, and religious holidays.

It's OK to eat—and enjoy—a small piece of cake with friends and family—especially if you scrape off most of the frosting.

132 Restaurant savvy I: Become a "regular."

Find a local restaurant you like and patronize it often. You'll get better, faster service—a blessing when your blood glucose is dropping. Having a regular waitperson also guarantees solicitous treatment: "This is fresh," or "This isn't as good today."

133 Restaurant savvy II: Always ask how a dish is made.

Then ask questions like:

"Can you serve it with the sauce on the side?"

"Can it be sauteed or stir-fried instead of fried?"

"Can the chef make it without flour or cornstarch? I don't care if the sauce is runny. Can it be made without starchy vegetables? With more mushrooms and peppers?"

134 Restaurant savvy III: Doggie-bag strategy.

Of course, given today's generous restaurant servings, you'll try to eat only half, and have the rest packed up for you in a doggie bag.

Realistically, though, many of us still get seduced into cleaning our plates. To avoid overeating, bring your own little covered plastic bowl and put half your entree into the bowl immediately. Then you can eat the rest and scrape your plate clean with a clear conscience.

135 Restaurant savvy IV: Order off the menu.

You can do this most easily if you're a regular at that restaurant.

At your local Chinese restaurant, for example, you can create your own dish:

"Can your chef mix breast of chicken with shrimp? In a brown sauce without flour or cornstarch? How about with shredded ginger? Tree ears? Black mushrooms? Sweet red and yellow peppers?"

At my local Chinese restaurant, I hand an index card to my waiter and ask him to show it to the chef. It has the English and Cantonese words for No Flour. No Sugar. No Cornstarch.

Be a Cantonese (or Szechuan) Escoffier! The sky's the limit, and your new creation will be loaded with vitamins and nutrients.

136 Restaurant savvy V: Bring restaurant ideas home.

Just as you bring your ideas to a favorite restaurant for execution, adapt a restaurant's dishes and presentations for home use.

It can be as simple as a garnish, or which fresh or dried herbs are used to embellish a dish. The unusual ingredients of a fresh fruit salad. Seasonings. (Many years later, I still remember the marvelous broiled grapefruit served at the former Chalet Suzanne in Lake Wales, Florida.)

Professional chefs have created these unusual dishes and presentations. Copying them can bring you compliments at home.

137 Got the munchies? Go for "fiddle" food.

"Fiddle" food is food that you have to fiddle with before you can eat it. You have to take it out of its shell, cut it up, unwrap it. That's going to slow down how much you eat. The best examples are nuts—especially almonds, walnuts, and Brazil nuts, which really take some work. *Bonus:* Unshelled nuts are also fresher and more nutritious. Unshelled pistachios will *really* slow you down.

Or try cutting up a whole fresh pineapple and nibbling on it instead of buying it already cut up.

138 Add nuts to main courses and salads.

When you add nuts to main courses and salads, you are also adding fiber and protein. For example, one ounce of walnuts contains three grams of carbohydrate and three grams of fiber—making 0 grams of net carbs—and five grams of protein.

Adding nuts adds texture too. You have to chew more, which increases the flavor and slows down your eating.

139 Navigate the carbohydrate controversy.

The American Diabetes Association's diet emphasizes carbohydrates. It urges us to get 50% to 60% of our calories from carbohydrates, which metabolize into sugars. The ADA website (Diabetes.org) tells us to make starches "the centerpiece of the meal."

The ADA is not alone in its advice. Boston's Joslin Diabetes Center recommends that 40% of our calories come from carbohydrates. Remember that each carb gram equals 4 calories. Here's a breakdown using the ADA's 55% yardstick:

CALORIES	CARBOHYDRATES	DAILY GRAMS BREAKFAST	LUNCH	DINNER	SNACK
1,200	166	33	58	58	17
1,500	206	41	72	72	21
1,800	248	50	87	87	25
2,100	289	58	101	101	29

Critics of these recommended high-carbohydrate diets are vocal. Among them are physicians who have diabetes. According to Richard Bernstein, MD, a type 1 diabetic for 70 years, people whose bodies can't process carbohydrates should not be told by the diabetic establishment to eat a diet that mostly metabolizes into sugar.

Admittedly, Dr. Bernstein's regimen is tough for many of us to follow. It limits carbohydrates to 6 grams for breakfast and 12 grams each for lunch and dinner—30 grams of carbohydrates per day. Nonetheless, many people with diabetes have had amazing success with it and have had normal test results for years.

Dr. Bernstein is not alone in his criticism. Diabetes specialist Lois Jovanovic, MD, calls the ADA high-carbohydrate diet "malpractice" because "diabetes is a disease of carbohydrate intolerance."

The Harvard School of Public Health found that the now-retired USDA "food pyramid"—"fats bad, carbohydrates good"—is "backward" and can actually increase the risk of heart attack, obesity, and stroke.

So how do *you* sort out the controversy? Logic seems to be on the side of Drs. Bernstein and Jovanovic and the Harvard Medical School. If you have gyrating blood-glucose readings and unacceptable lab results, consider trying to restrict your daily carbohydrates to 30 grams or, if that's too difficult, to 60 grams for one month. Remember to use *net* carbohydrates. If you and your doctor are happy with the results, stay with your new low-carbohydrate eating plan.

140 For pizza lovers.

Don't give up your favorite pizza, just ditch the dough. Even thin-crust pizzas can contain 10 to 15 grams of carbohydrate per slice in the crust.

Pick up your fork and enjoy the pizza topping, which has much more flavor and protein. You can probably have two slices' worth if you skip the crust.

141 Enjoy the crunch of raw food.

There's a serious kick in foods with texture. In addition to carrot and celery sticks, try strips of sweet peppers, green beans, and even asparagus stalks.

Explore the dozens of varieties of pears developed specifically for eating, rather than cooking. A piece of fruit and a wedge of cheese can make an easy, nutritious meal.

142 Burn calories with ice water.

Drinking ice water has a benefit beyond hydrating you and cooling you off. Your body must burn calories to bring the ice water up to your body temperature—as much as 200 calories per day.

143 Buy at farm stands and farmers' markets.

For freshness and variety, farm stands and farmers' markets are your best bets. Many neighborhoods in large cities now offer farmers' markets at least once a week.

Farms and orchards where you can pick your own berries and fruits are another great choice. The bending and stretching will also exercise you, and picking berries and fruits is a wonderful education for your children and grandchildren.

144 Grow your own.

Better yet, grow your own! Even if all you have is a kitchen window, you can grow your own herbs. Rosemary, basil, and tarragon are good choices.

Need more room? A planter on a terrace, a backyard patch, or a little piece of a community garden will give you enough room for at least one or two raspberry bushes, encircled by strawberry plants. (Gardeners call this doubling-up tactic "underplanting." It lets you utilize every square inch of space.) Tomatoes need lots of depth for their roots, but you can usually grow patio tomatoes in a planter, or even a plastic wastebasket with holes drilled in the bottom for drainage.

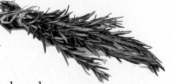

More space in warmer climates will let you grow vegetables and fruit trees.

Photo: Creadtiveye99

Nothing is more fun than picking your own food and eating it right away! When autumns are mild, I've grown and picked my own raspberries and tomatoes as late as Thanksgiving.

145 Go garlic!

Many of us feel that garlic should be elevated to its own food group. Besides tasting marvelous and being the soul food of many ethnic groups, garlic has many medical benefits. It lowers blood pressure and is an anticoagulant and a powerful antibiotic. It also boosts the immune system.

146 "Sugar-free" is not carbohydrate-free.

You probably already know that high-fructose corn syrup and glucose—two common ingredients in processed foods—are not considered "sugar" for the purposes of food labeling, but can drive your blood glucose into the stratosphere. Honey isn't as common an ingredient because it's much more expensive.

Sugar alcohols—ingredients that end in "itol," like maltitol—are ingredients that many people with diabetes are not as familiar with. Most of them discover that sugar alcohol makes their blood-glucose levels zoom, so they learn to read food labels carefully and avoid foods made with it.

147 The benefits of breakfast.

Your mother was right. Breakfast is the most important meal of the day. Your body has been without food for approximately 12 hours, which means that your rate of burning calories has slowed down. If you make lunch your first meal, then your metabolic rate has dropped for 18 hours. Harvard Medical School researchers found that breakfast eaters have one-half the risk of developing obesity and insulin resistance, which is a major risk factor for diabetes and heart disease, compared with people who skip breakfast.

Other studies show that people who eat breakfast eat less fat and fewer high-calorie foods all day. They are also less likely to overeat at night.

148 Breakfast on the go.

You can make yourself a low-calorie grab-and-go breakfast in less than five minutes.

Put 1 cup of plain lowfat yogurt in a small container. If desired, mix in one or two teaspoons of fruit spread or frozen berries.

Or take a small wedge of your favorite cheese or ½ cup of lowfat cottage cheese. Add an apple or an orange and a travel mug of coffee or tea. Now you can breakfast at your desk.

149 Salad dressing smarts I: The small-portion solution.

According to the labels on the bottles, two tablespoons constitutes a portion. That means horrendously high calorie, carbohydrate, and fat counts—often 160 to 170 calories per portion, which equals 10% of many diabetics' daily allowance.

However, you can cut back on that two-tablespoon portion easily. If you limit yourself to one to two *teaspoons* of your favorite salad dressing, you'll be consuming only 17% to 33% of those calories, carbohydrates, and fats.

150 Salad dressing smarts II: Pour off the oil.

Many bottled salad dressings are made with oil that rises to the top. Cut the calories and fat and intensify the flavor by pouring off at least half the oil as soon as you open the bottle. Then refrigerate, of course.

151 Salad dressing smarts III: Dilute the fat and calories.

If your favorite salad dressing is a ranch or creamy type, dilute it with an equal quantity of lowfat buttermilk.

You'll still have the zesty flavor, but you'll cut the calories and fat.

152 Salad dressing smarts IV: Skinny-dip!

What's a salad without dressing? Boring, and possibly even tasteless. To solve this problem, when you get your low-calorie, low-fat salad dressing on the side, dip your fork into the dressing before spearing the greens. You'll use a lot less dressing this way, so you'll get almost all the taste, but avoid almost all the calories and fat.

153 Beefy bonus.

You can feel good about eating beef. Lean beef packs a powerful nutritional punch. Ounce for ounce, it delivers three times more iron, six times more zinc, and eight times more vitamin B-12 than a skinless chicken breast.

154 Feast on homemade nut butters.

Do you love peanut butter but want to avoid those nasty hydrogenated oils? Make your own!

All you need is a blender or food processor, dry-roasted or raw unsalted peanuts, and about five minutes. Blend until crunchy or smooth.

You can also make almond or cashew butter with raw nuts, or toast them first in the oven.

Once you make nut butters at home, you'll never want supermarket peanut butter again.

155 Make your own no-carbohydrate maple syrup.

Many people with diabetes miss having maple syrup on their weekend low-carbohydrate French toast or pancakes. The real thing is too high in carbohydrates and calories and can wreck your blood glucose numbers.

Instead, use maple extract straight from the bottle. Dilute it with water. Add Equal if it's not sweet enough. Pour and enjoy!

156 Keep fat in your diet.

There are many good reasons to keep some fat in your diet.

Fat causes your body to produce the smallest amount of insulin. Replacing dietary fat with carbohydrates actually causes higher insulin levels, and that will increase your body fat and can lead to obesity.

Fat also stops carbohydrate cravings. It satisfies our hunger longer, so we are less tempted to eat. A few grams of fat per day can wind up saving hundreds of calories a day in food intake.

And a little fat in your diet makes your skin glow—especially as you grow older.

157 Start your diet on Saturday.

We're all familiar with the "I'll start my diet on Monday" syndrome. The problem is that we then act like condemned criminals facing their last meals and pig out. After all, we'll start a strict diet tomorrow.

The result is that we lose two days and usually put on five pounds. And we start the week beating up on ourselves and feeling guilty.

Saturday can be an easier day to start your diet. You are usually not as rushed and can linger over a well-planned breakfast, lunch, and dinner. You can even do some gourmet cooking for the rest of the week.

By Monday, you will have gotten a head start on your diet. And you'll probably weigh less, too.

158 Ice cream calories and carbohydrates vary greatly.

Ice cream calories and carbohydrates can vary by more than 100% per portion. For example, a half-cup portion of Breyer's coffee ice cream has 140 calories and 14 grams of carbohydrate, easy for diabetics and dieters alike to fit into their meal plans. But the same size portion of superpremium Godiva Chocolate Raspberry Truffle ice cream contains 290 calories and 32 grams of carbohydrate, which can really capsize your diet.

159 Understand your emotional eating.

Many people eat for reasons that have nothing to do with physical hunger. They may be angry, anxious, bored, lonely, or sad.

It's not easy, and it can be painful, but try to find the reason you are eating (usually overeating) and deal with it. Confide your feelings to a journal, then call a friend or go for a walk, rent a movie, or tune in to the Cartoon Network or Comedy Central.

160 Dieting? Atkins may work better than other plans.

Multiple studies have found that people on low-carbohydrate diets, like the Atkins plan, ate more than those on an American Heart Association lowfat diet—and still lost weight. The no-carb life is not forever, but it can give you a head start.

This news comes as no surprise to many of us diabetic patients who thrive on limiting our carbohydrates rather than counting every single calorie.

161 Customize your weight-loss plan.

In dieting, one size does not fit all. We all have our favorite foods and hated foods, carbohydrate foods that raise our blood-glucose readings horrendously and those that don't. Some of us fare better on three meals a day, and some with four or five smaller meals.

Find a plan that works for *you*. It may take weeks of trial and error, but what counts is *your* long-term success in losing weight and keeping it off.

162 Work your favorite foods into your weight-loss plan.

You can prevent binge eating by including your favorite foods in your weight-loss or eating plan.

One of my diabetic friends, who is a diabetes educator, says, "I'll work out at the gym in order to have ice cream." Most of us would agree.

Even without the workout, you can plan for a small dish of ice cream or two small pieces of chocolate or a piece of fruit for dessert every night without exceeding your carbohydrate quota. And that little treat can satisfy you enough to keep you on your diet the rest of the time.

163 Substitute spray for shortening.

Do the math and you'll become a convert.

One tablespoon of oil contains 122 calories, one tablespoon of butter or margarine, 104 calories. But a one-second spritz of cooking spray—enough to coat an omelet pan or skillet—contains only seven calories.

Cooking sprays come in several flavors, like butter, olive oil, and garlic.

164 Don't fool yourself into rationalizing portion size.

Yes, those little ice-cream cups cost more per serving than a 48-ounce container of ice cream; but yes, there's a built-in portion-control factor with those little cardboard cups. An open container of ice cream with no markings for servings is a hollering temptation to stick your spoon back in again…and again. If your frugal soul chafes at the cost-per-ounce of the individual-serving cups, consider that a portion of the cost actually goes to limiting your consumption; part of your purchase price is the built-in self-control. You can eat the whole thing and scrape out that little cup, and that "extra cost" is actually an investment well spent.

165 Artificial sweeteners can increase appetite and weight gain.

No, it's not what you were hoping and praying for, but here's the science behind it.

This is how it works: A study published in the July 12, 2016, issue of *Cell Metabolism* found that "after chronic exposure to a diet that contained the artificial sweetener sucralose, we saw that animals began eating a lot more." And therefore the weight gain.

And here's how you can fight it: Substitute cinnamon or small pieces of fruit for those sweeteners. Better yet, learn to relish the taste of unsweetened food. Your palate will thank you!

166 Understand the BMI.

The Body Mass Index (BMI) is a convenient number that expresses the ratio of your weight to your height as a single number.

To calculate it, multiply your weight in pounds by 703. Divide this number by your height in inches, and then divide it again by your height in inches. (Or just Google "BMI calculator" and input the data in an online calculator.)

Body Mass Index Table 1

BMI	19	20	21	22	23	24	25	26	27	28	29	30	31	32	33	34	35
Height (inches)	Body Weight (pounds)																
58	91	96	100	105	110	115	119	124	129	134	138	143	148	153	158	162	167
59	94	99	104	109	114	119	124	128	133	138	143	148	153	158	163	168	173
60	97	102	107	112	118	123	128	133	138	143	148	153	158	163	168	174	179
61	100	106	111	116	122	127	132	137	143	148	153	158	164	169	174	180	185
62	104	109	115	120	126	131	136	142	147	153	158	164	169	175	180	186	191
63	107	113	118	124	130	135	141	146	152	158	163	169	175	180	186	191	197
64	110	116	122	128	134	140	145	151	157	163	169	174	180	186	192	197	204
65	114	120	126	132	138	144	150	156	162	168	174	180	186	192	198	204	210
66	118	124	130	136	142	148	155	161	167	173	179	186	192	198	204	210	216
67	121	127	134	140	146	153	159	166	172	178	185	191	198	204	211	217	223
68	125	131	138	144	151	158	164	171	177	184	190	197	203	210	216	223	230
69	128	135	142	149	155	162	169	176	182	189	196	203	209	216	223	230	236
70	132	139	146	153	160	167	174	181	188	195	202	209	216	222	229	236	243
71	136	143	150	157	165	172	179	186	193	200	208	215	222	229	236	243	250
72	140	147	154	162	169	177	184	191	199	206	213	221	228	235	242	250	258
73	144	151	159	166	174	182	189	197	204	212	219	227	235	242	250	257	265
74	148	155	163	171	179	186	194	202	210	218	225	233	241	249	256	264	272
75	152	160	168	176	184	192	200	208	216	224	232	240	248	256	264	272	279
76	156	164	172	180	189	197	205	213	221	230	238	246	254	263	271	279	287

Body Mass Index Table 2

BMI	36	37	38	39	40	41	42	43	44	45	46	47	48	49	50	51	52	53	54
Height (inches)	Body Weight (pounds)																		
58	172	177	181	186	191	196	201	205	210	215	220	224	229	234	239	244	248	253	258
59	178	183	188	193	198	203	208	212	217	222	227	232	237	242	247	252	257	262	267
60	184	189	194	199	204	209	215	220	225	230	235	240	245	250	255	261	266	271	276
61	190	195	201	206	211	217	222	227	232	238	243	248	254	259	264	269	275	280	285
62	196	202	207	213	218	224	229	235	240	246	251	256	262	267	273	278	284	289	295
63	203	208	214	220	225	231	237	242	248	254	259	265	270	278	282	287	293	299	304
64	209	215	221	227	232	238	244	250	256	262	267	273	279	285	291	296	302	308	314
65	216	222	228	234	240	246	252	258	264	270	276	282	288	294	300	306	312	318	324
66	223	229	235	241	247	253	260	266	272	278	284	291	297	303	309	315	322	328	334
67	230	236	242	249	255	261	268	274	280	287	293	299	306	312	319	325	331	338	344
68	236	243	249	256	262	269	276	282	289	295	302	308	315	322	328	335	341	348	354
69	243	250	257	263	270	277	284	291	297	304	311	318	324	331	338	345	351	358	365
70	250	257	264	271	278	285	292	299	306	313	320	327	334	341	348	355	362	369	376
71	257	265	272	279	286	293	301	308	315	322	329	338	343	351	358	365	372	379	386
72	265	272	279	287	294	302	309	316	324	331	338	346	353	361	368	375	383	390	397
73	272	280	288	295	302	310	318	325	333	340	348	355	363	371	378	386	393	401	408
74	280	287	295	303	311	319	326	334	342	350	358	365	373	381	389	396	404	412	420
75	287	295	303	311	319	327	335	343	351	359	367	375	383	391	399	407	415	423	431
76	295	304	312	320	328	336	344	353	361	369	377	385	394	402	410	418	426	435	443

Thus, someone who is 5'5" tall and weighs 160 pounds has a BMI of 26.6. A BMI under 18.5 is considered underweight, 18.5-24.9 is considered normal, 25.0-29.9 is considered overweight, and over 30.0 is considered obese.

However, there are limitations to this easy-to-understand number. The most common is that serious bodybuilders may have BMIs between 25 and 30, but not be overweight because muscle tissue weighs more than fat.

167 Enjoy your wine!

You may have heard of "the French paradox," which suggests that the French consumption of wine offsets the fat in their diet and helps prevent coronary disease and cancer.

Here's the science behind it: Wine—especially red wine—contains large quantities of resveratrol, a phytochemical that has been linked to a reduced risk of coronary disease and cancer. Some plants, fruits, seeds, and other grape products contain resveratrol, too, but not in as high a concentration, and many of them are high in carbohydrates.

A glass of dry red wine at dinner offers other benefits, including increasing HDL (good) cholesterol in some people.

There's very little difference in calories or carbohydrates (both minimal) among the different varieties of dry red wine, so just choose your favorite!

168 Cook with it, too.

Cooking with wine adds flavor, but not calories. That's because heat evaporates the alcohol, leaving only the wonderful taste.

The increased flavor also lets you reduce less beneficial ingredients, like fat or oil and salt.

Cooking with liquors like cognac, rum, or bourbon doesn't add calories either, but sweet liqueurs like amaretto and Grand Marnier should be used sparingly because of their high caloric and carbohydrate content.

169 Jump-start your diet with a fast.

Admittedly, this strategy isn't for everyone, but a one- or two-day fast drinking only water won't hurt most adults and should pay off in a weight loss of approximately five pounds.

Please check first with your doctor.

You must also…

Drink at least six 8-ounce glasses of water per day.

Adjust your insulin so that you are taking only your long-acting, basal dosage, not the dose or type of insulin you need for meal coverage.

170 Could a "starvation diet" cure type 2 diabetes? Maybe.

In a Newcastle (UK) University study published in *Diabetes Care* in March 2016, researchers gave type 2 diabetes patients an eight-week very-low-calorie diet limited to three diet milkshakes and approximately seven ounces of vegetables a day. The patients lost an average of about 31 pounds, and half of them lost their diabetes symptoms for six months after returning to their usual diets.

171 Check package labels for trans fats.

On June 16, 2015, the FDA finalized its determination that trans fats are not "generally recognized as safe" and ordered a three-year time limit (June 18, 2018) for their removal from all processed foods.

My advice: Don't buy foods containing trans fats *now*. Check the label.

172 Make cottage cheese more exciting.

Lovely, bland cottage cheese is a dieter's friend. (But it's not always a diabetic person's friend.) Diabetes specialist and long-term diabetic Dr. Richard Bernstein says it increases blood glucose a lot in some of his patients. One trick to reduce the lactose content is to rinse the cottage cheese before you use it. The 2% fat variety contains 90 calories, 6 grams of carbohydrate, 2.5 grams of fat, and 12 grams of protein per ½-cup serving, and the 1% variety contains only 80 calories, 4 grams of carbohydrate, 1 gram of fat, and 14 grams of protein.

But this diet standby can get a little boring after a while.

Go spicy or sweet to perk up your interest without boosting your calorie or carbohydrate intake.

Spicy: Add freeze-dried chives or onions (nice and crunchy!), garlic powder, chopped hot or sweet peppers, a teaspoon of salad dressing, salsa, or mustard.

Sweet: Add vanilla, almond, orange, lemon, or peppermint extract, with or without sugar substitute.

173 Make sure you get enough protein.

With all the emphasis on carbohydrates by diabetic patients and their doctors, protein is often neglected. But many patients don't get enough protein every day, and their doctors don't point out how crucial it is.

Protein is the building block of the body. Without enough protein, your body will start breaking down to nourish itself.

How much is enough? A simple rule of thumb is one-half gram of protein for every pound you weigh. For example, a 150-pound person should consume 75 grams of protein a day, with approximately one-third at each meal. It's OK to eat more protein unless you have kidney disease, but don't eat less.

174 Eat spinach at least three times a week.

Spinach can help prevent two eye diseases that diabetic patients are especially susceptible to: cataracts and age-related macular degeneration.

Spinach is loaded with folate and the phytochemicals lutein and zeaxanthin, both of which are found in the macula (central portion) of the retina. Zeaxanthin has been linked to a lower risk of age-related macular degeneration, the leading cause of blindness in people over the age of 55. Zeaxanthin is also believed to protect against the development of cataracts.

Maybe Popeye was right!

Note: Orange peppers also have a high zeaxanthin and lutein content, but they are seasonal and often expensive.

175 Weight-y matters.

It makes more sense to weigh yourself once a week than every single day.

Even if you weigh yourself at the same time every morning (after the bathroom and before breakfast), your weight can still fluctuate by two to three pounds from day to day.

If you weigh yourself only once a week, these little increases and decreases smooth out, and you get a more accurate reading and sense of your progress.

However, if you are obsessive and *must* weigh yourself every morning, keep track of your daily numbers in a notebook and divide by seven once a week to calculate your average weight.

176 Substitute spaghetti squash for pasta.

Plain pasta is high in carbohydrates, the bane of many people with diabetes. One cup of cooked regular or whole-wheat pasta, for example, contains approximately 198 calories and 41 grams of carbohydrate. But one cup of spaghetti squash contains only 46 calories and 10 grams of carbohydrate. Spaghetti squash is also an excellent source of folic acid and fiber and contributes some potassium and a small amount of vitamin A.

Mangia!

177 When you *must* bake.

Sometimes we all get the urge to bake. It's OK to give in to that warm, nurturing desire if you plan ahead to prevent potential binge eating. *Here's what you can do…*

Invite one or more friends for coffee and that fresh-baked goodie. Give them any leftovers to take home.

Eat one and freeze the rest for future feasting.

Or eat one and bring the rest to an older neighbor or to a nursing home.

178 Cinnamon bun substitute.

Breakfast pastries have been supersized to mammoth proportions. A Cinnabon cinnamon roll weighs 7½ ounces and contains 880 calories—nearly half the daily allowance for most of us—with 58 grams of sugar and 37 grams of fat. Their Caramel Pecanbon is even worse: 1,080 calories and 51 grams of fat.

But you can get a cinnamon-bun taste without all the calories, carbohydrates, and fat.

Take a slice of whole-wheat or whole-grain bread, spread with a thin layer of butter or margarine, sprinkle with cinnamon and a sugar substitute. Warm in the microwave and eat. Total calories approximately 100, with 13 grams of carbohydrate and less than 3 grams of fat. Using thin-sliced bread? Cut these numbers in half.

179 Cinnamon boosts the effects of insulin.

Just one-quarter teaspoon of cinnamon increases the effect of insulin that your body produces or that you inject. Scientists at the USDA Human Nutrition Research Center discovered that methylhydroxy chalcone polymer (MHCP)—the active chemical in cinnamon—makes insulin 20 times more active.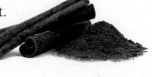

Photo: eyewave

According to a study published in the November 2015 issue of *Today's Dietitian*, cinnamon improves blood glucose, triglycerides, total cholesterol, and HDL and LDL cholesterol levels in type 2 diabetics when they consume as little as 6 grams of cinnamon daily.

No studies to date show a benefit of using cinnamon in type 1 diabetes because it is an autoimmune disease and cinnamon can't restore insulin production in pancreatic beta cells once they have been destroyed.

Conclusion: If you have type 2 diabetes, adding cinnamon to your food intake will probably produce the good results mentioned in the journal article. If you are a type 1 diabetic, as I am, add cinnamon to your daily diet for the cardiovascular and cholesterol benefits. I've been adding cinnamon to my daily breakfast for about 20 years. And it tastes so good!

180 There's cinnamon...and cinnamon.

Not all cinnamons are created equal. Cinnamaldehyde, the active chemical, helps reduce insulin resistance by increasing glucose uptake in the body. But spice-rack cinnamons vary widely in their amounts of cinnamaldehyde, so check with your doctor for a brand recommendation. Cinnamon capsules are produced by many vitamin manufacturers, or you can make your own if you're handy. You can buy empty capsules for filling at most pharmacies.

Make sure that cinnamon doesn't react negatively with any drugs you are taking.

181 Other herbs and spices work, too.

Allspice, nutmeg, and oregano also make insulin more potent. They increase the effect of insulin more than eight times.

Of these, oregano is the least expensive and the easiest to add to your daily menu. It goes well with fresh tomatoes and tomato sauces, and it is easy to grow on your windowsill or in a small herb garden.

182 Turmeric may prevent—even reverse—type 1 and type 2 diabetes.

Turmeric, a plant of the ginger family, is grown and used throughout Southeast Asia to treat many medical problems. It is currently being studied for its potential to affect many diseases, including kidney and cardiovascular diseases, arthritis, cancer, and diabetes. Many diabetic patients are not waiting for these studies and are adding turmeric to their daily diets.

183 Yo-yo dieting is harmful.

You lose weight. You gain it back. You lose weight. You gain it back. This time it's harder to lose the weight, and you may gain back even more, and more quickly.

This repeated pattern, called "yo-yo dieting," is dangerous. In its infinite wisdom, your body senses each successive diet as an attempt to starve it. Your body defends itself by slowing down your metabolism. Your body will actually try to increase its fat deposits to protect itself, and this can lead to cardiovascular disease and stroke.

184 How to deal with your "thrifty gene."

The "thrifty gene" theory explains our species' survival in the face of famine and disease. Historically, many population groups have survived times when food was scarce and uncertain because some of them were able to slow down their metabolism and live on very few calories. Those people lived to pass on their "thrifty gene" to successive generations. It is Darwin's "survival of the fittest" in action.

Fast-forward to the present. Rather than hunting and gathering or growing our own food and fearing famine, most of our hunting is for the nearest parking space in the supermarket lot. Now food is readily available, but our genes haven't learned that.

By adolescence or young adulthood, most of us know whether we possess the thrifty gene. We have learned through bitter experience how difficult it is for us to lose even five or 10 pounds while our friends brag how much they can eat without gaining weight.

How do you deal with your thrifty gene? Try these three strategies:

First, bring balance and sanity into your life by recognizing that you have a thrifty gene. You may never become an athlete or wear a size 4, but you should survive the next famine or Ice Age.

Second, avoid gaining any more weight. Lose weight slowly—over years, not weeks. Crash dieting will only make your thrifty gene more thrifty.

Third, increase your activity level. Try the tips in Chapter 5, "Exercise."

185 Snacks can help you lose weight.

You may be more successful with an eating plan that offers a midmorning and a midafternoon snack. The logic is that you will not overeat at meals and so will actually eat less overall.

Typical "good" snacks are skinless turkey or chicken, low-fat cheese, hard-boiled eggs, vegetables, and small quantities of fresh fruit.

186 Indulge in the hot stuff.

Your love of spicy food can help you lose weight. In a study published in *British Journal of Nutrition* in 1999, researchers found that when people ate a red sauce made with capsaicin—the phytochemical that makes chili peppers hot—they ate 200 fewer calories over the next three hours than when the sauce did not contain capsaicin.

Even better, in a large study reported in January 13, 2017, *Science News*, University of Vermont Langner College of Medicine researchers found that consumption of hot red chili peppers was associated with a 13% reduction in total mortality, primarily in deaths from cardiovascular disease or stroke. The study was published in *PLOS ONE*.

187 Know your dieting style.

Do you prefer to weigh or measure your food? To count calories or carbohydrates? To eat meals or to graze? The closer your dieting plan comes to matching your usual eating pattern, the more likely it is that you will stick to your diet and lose weight.

188 Give yourself "wiggle room."

Whether or not you are dieting, your weight fluctuates every day. A range of three to five pounds is quite normal.

Give yourself some leeway. Don't be concerned as long as your weight stays within that five-pound range. But if your weight rises above that limit, it's time to diet more seriously.

189 Belts beat scales.

Dieting? Is the needle on your scale stuck? Try on a belt. Sometimes it takes a week or two before your scale shows a weight loss. But during that time your waistline will start shrinking, and your belt will demonstrate that it has.

Keep on using that belt to check your progress. Especially when your weight hits a plateau and you become depressed, having to cinch your belt tighter will show you that your diet is really working.

190 Knit or crochet.

Why is this tip in this chapter? Because knitting and crocheting can help you lose weight. Not only do they keep your fingers busy and away from food, but the clicking of the knitting needles and the in-and-out movement of the crochet hook are repetitive actions that can soothe you and send you into another, relaxing "zone."

Football great Rosey Grier made it acceptable for men to do needlepoint, so why shouldn't they try knitting or crocheting? A scarf is a great beginner's project because it needs no shaping and its finished measurements can be off by several inches and it won't be obvious.

191 Salad-bar pitfalls.

Salad bars can be perilous. The greens are great, but portion control and avoiding all the add-ons can be a problem. Steer clear of bacon chips, croutons, the dressings, some of which are loaded with calories, and the crackers and bread that are often served with them.

If you like the convenience and variety that salad bars offer, load up on the greens and raw vegetables, and spoon out the dressing parsimoniously.

192 Brown-bag your lunch.

When you bring your lunch from home, you are lured less by the ubiquitous fast-food restaurants and takeouts, and by nearby candy and soda machines.

Go gourmet with your own mixture of lowfat plain yogurt and diced fresh fruit or berries. Make salmon, crabmeat, or shrimp salad the night before, or eat the seafood unadorned, out of the can. Eat raw veggies as finger food, with or without a *teaspoon* of salad dressing. (You can be more lavish with mustard.)

193 Break your binge.

Even the most dedicated dieter is bound to binge once every few months. Here are some ways to deal with this problem:

If you really, truly binge only once in a very great while, give yourself permission to do so, and adjust your medication—if necessary—the next time you check your blood glucose. *But* be honest with yourself about how often this behavior occurs. Set a kitchen timer for five or 10 minutes and *stop eating when the bell rings.*

If you binge more frequently, be aware of what triggers this behavior. The simplest fix is removing yourself from the "scene of the crime." Get out of your house and go for a walk. Visit a friend.

A stronger strategy comes from practitioners of aversion therapy. Place a thick rubber band over your wrist. It should fit snugly, like a bracelet. When you find yourself bingeing, snap the rubber band on the underside of your wrist—it should hurt—and say "Stop!" to yourself. Repeat if necessary.

194 Underdressing burns more calories.

Dress in lighter clothes than you need—you should feel a little cold, but not uncomfortably so—and your body thermostat has to work harder to maintain your temperature. That means burning more calories—about 5% more. You may also move more briskly to keep warm, and that will burn even more calories.

195 Apple pie substitute I.

Sauteed apples can satisfy your taste for apple pie. But where a slice of apple pie contains 405 calories, 60 grams of carbohydrate, and 18 grams of fat, a three-ounce "snack pie" contains 266 calories, 33 grams of carbohydrate, and 14 grams of fat. This recipe, which I created, contains only between 80 and 100 calories (depending on the size of the apple), 21 grams of carbohydrate, and less than two grams of fat—scarcely more than a raw apple.

For each serving, peel and core one apple and cut it into eight to 10 pieces. Spray a large skillet heavily with butter-flavored cooking spray and, if desired, 1 teaspoon butter. Add apple, stir, turn heat down, cover, and cook for 10 minutes. Sprinkle with 1 tablespoon sugar substitute and 1 teaspoon cinnamon. Raise heat to medium. Cook, stirring frequently, until apple pieces are glazed—approximately 10 minutes. Serve hot or warm.

196 Apple pie substitute II.

Baked apples are another tasty treat. This recipe, too, contains only about 20 calories more than a raw apple.

Preheat oven to 350 degrees. For each serving, take a large apple and core and peel the top half, leaving the bottom half intact. Dip the peeled portion into a mixture of one tablespoon lemon juice and 10 tablespoons water to prevent browning.

Place the apple in a baking dish with approximately one-half inch of water at the bottom. Dilute ½ teaspoon no-sugar-added raspberry or apricot fruit spread with ½ teaspoon of water and spread on top of apple. Bake approximately 40 minutes.

Then fill the cavity of the apple with one teaspoon of the fruit spread and bake an additional 10 minutes. Serve hot or warm.

197 Lighten your beer.

The new "lite" and "ultralite" beers are a godsend to people with diabetes who love their brew. New brewing technologies have kept the flavor, but cut the calories and carbohydrates by one-third to one-half. Brewers will certainly keep on making their beers and ales more attractive to dieters, so keep on checking labels and websites for the latest new drinkables.

198 Know your yogurts.

This is a food in which calorie, carbohydrate, protein, and fiber counts vary dramatically. To add to the confusion, some yogurts have all kinds of other ingredients included or packaged as an add-on, and some plain varieties are made of skim milk, while some are made of whole milk.

After examining 40 or 50 labels, there's only one type of yogurt that I'd eat because it's the only one with any fiber: Chobani Simply 100. One container has 100 calories, 10 grams of protein, and 3 grams of fiber in various flavors, giving people who eat two containers 20 grams of protein and six grams of fiber in 200 calories. With a snack added, it's still a low-calorie lunch!

199 Use yogurt cheese instead of cream cheese.

You'll need a little advance planning (like the night before), a funnel, and a coffee filter. Your reward is a freshly made cheese that can be used like cream cheese or Neufchatel, with only a fraction of the calories and fat.

Preparation takes less than three minutes. Place the coffee filter in the funnel and suspend it in a glass or small bowl. Then fill the filter with plain lowfat yogurt, cover it with plastic wrap, and refrigerate overnight. Discard the whey (liquid). Use the resulting cheese au naturel, blend fresh or dried herbs and garlic into it, or add vanilla or other flavoring extracts. Or you can substitute it for cream cheese in recipes.

Here's the caloric breakdown: Two ounces of regular or whipped cream cheese contains 200 calories, two grams of carbohydrate, 20 grams of fat, and four grams of protein. Calculating the calories, carbohydrates, and fat content of yogurt cheese is a little less precise because of the speed at which the whey drains out of the yogurt and because there are no calculations for the whey itself.

However, the equivalent one-quarter cup of plain low-fat yogurt contains only 35 calories, four grams of fat, and 2.7 grams of protein. Furthermore, the whey, which is discarded, is a rich source of lactose (milk sugar), so the yogurt cheese you make probably contains less than 1 gram of carbohydrate.

200 Be honest with yourself.

Recently I ran into an acquaintance and was shocked to see that he had gained 30 pounds (about 20% of his body weight) in less than a year. When I asked him what had happened, he told me that he was now driving a cab 12 hours a day and living on fast food, like buying and devouring three hamburgers one after the other, or a box of doughnuts, or a pizza.

"Why don't you buy five or six burgers and eat the meat and toss the buns?" I asked him.

"Well, I can't," he answered evasively.

"Why don't you bring cheese slices and a couple of apples from home? You can eat lots of good food with one hand."

He didn't have a good answer for that, either.

He wasn't being honest with me, and I doubt that he is honest with himself. That will be his first step in planning to lose weight.

201 Fast-food restaurants may be worth a second look.

After too many years, fast-food restaurants are finally offering low-carbohydrate, low-fat dishes that we can eat. Chains like Applebee's, Burger King, McDonald's, Ruby Tuesday, and Wendy's have all added grilled chicken, main-course salads, steamed vegetables, and other nutritious entrees to boost their business among health-conscious consumers. These good-for-you choices are usually highlighted or starred, which makes their menus easier to navigate.

202 Choose your bread wisely.

Most varieties of bread contain approximately the same number of calories and grams of carbohydrate per slice. But their glycemic index can differ greatly, which means that some varieties will not make your blood glucose zoom as much as others will.

The fineness or coarseness of the flour and the bread make a difference in how rapidly your body breaks down the bread into glucose. The best breads for us diabetics are made of oats (kernels or bran) or rye. Rye, which includes pumpernickel, is especially nutritious, as it contains more protein, phosphorus, iron, potassium, B vitamins, and 3.5 times as much soluble fiber as wheat bread. Sourdough rye bread has one of the lowest glycemic-index and glycemic-load values of all breads.

Although bread in general has gotten much more nutritious over the past 20 years, there are still huge differences among breads.

Among white breads, a slice of Arnold Brick Oven Premium White weighs 33 grams and contains 80 calories and 16 grams of carbohydrate, less than one gram of fiber and two grams of protein. A slice of Pepperidge Farm Hearty white bread weighs a heftier 43 grams and contains 110 calories and 20 grams of carbohydrate, one gram of fiber, and four grams of protein.

But compare this to a California-produced sprouted flaxseed bread. Two thin slices weigh 45 grams, contain 100 calories, 18 grams of carbohydrate, five grams of fiber (only 13 net grams of carbohydrate), and six grams of protein.

Photo: SednevaAnna

Flaxseed, the star of this bread, can also help osteoarthritis patients. According to a May 4, 2016, article in *Arthritis Today*, two tablespoons of ground flaxseed contain over 140% of the daily value of omega-3 fatty acids and more lignans, a cancer-fighting phytochemical, than any other plant food. The article also points out that flaxseed is an excellent source of fiber.

203 Adding acid can lower your blood glucose.

Researchers have found that a small amount of lemon juice or vinegar as an ingredient in salad dressing lowered blood glucose significantly. As little as six teaspoons of vinaigrette (four teaspoons vinegar, two teaspoons oil) eaten in a salad at lunch or dinner lowered blood glucose by as much as 30%.

Lemon juice was found to be just as effective, so consider a glass or two of homemade cold or hot lemonade (sweetened with a sugar substitute, of course).

204 Grisly fantasies may motivate you to lose weight.

Some people are more motivated by rewards, some by the possibility of punishment. If you respond more to the latter, think of the terrible things that can happen to you if you do not lose your excess weight and control your blood glucose better.

The possibility of having toes, feet, or legs amputated, of going blind, of needing a kidney transplant or going on dialysis may be frightening enough to make you decide to take action to improve your health.

205 Dieter's mantra.

When you are considering eating something, ask yourself: "Is this really worth all the calories, carbohydrates, and fat?" Reciting this mantra will give you perspective:

"A minute on my lips, a year on my hips."

206 No-carbohydrate lunches boost afternoon alertness.

Eating a no-carbohydrate lunch of lean meat or fish and salad or green vegetables helps you avoid the common afternoon slump. Here's why it works: Cutting carbohydrates prevents the release of serotonin, a brain chemical that can relax you to the point of sleep. But protein raises your level of dopamine, a brain chemical that boosts your alertness and also produces feelings of intense well-being.

207 Find a diet buddy.

A friendly sense of competition can help both you and a friend lose weight.

Choose the same morning of the week to strip down to your skivvies and weigh in. Keep track of your starting weights in a small notebook, and use the same scale every week for consistency. Bet no more than $5 or $10 per week, and the winner is the one who has lost the greatest percentage of weight that week. Keep up this little contest for at least 10 weeks, and you'll both be winners!

208 Belt up before you party.

Are you going to a party where there will be lots of food and drink? Make a belt part of your outfit and cinch it snugly, or wear it under your clothing. Your suddenly tight belt will tell you that you couldn't—or shouldn't—eat another bite.

209 Get nutty I.

Unsalted nuts are good for you! They are rich in protein, minerals, fiber, B vitamins including folic acid, vitamin E, and healthful monounsaturated fats. Walnuts are especially rich in these good oils, but almonds contain nearly three times as much fiber. Pistachios and cashews are good choices, too.

210 A daily egg can be safe.

The bad news: One egg contains 215 milligram of cholesterol, two-thirds of the daily maximum.

The good news: Saturated fat plays a larger role in raising our blood cholesterol, and eggs contain very little saturated fat. So if your cholesterol is low and you are not at risk for heart disease, you can probably enjoy a daily egg, low in calories and high in protein and iron.

Free-range eggs often offer better nutritional value.

Note: The Harvard School of Public Health website (www.hsph.harvard.edu) advises people with diabetes to have no more than three egg yolks per week. Consider cooking liquid egg substitute or egg whites if you want eggs more often.

211 Butter? Margarine?

Margarine that is made from hydrogenated oil contains trans fats, which are worse for your heart than the saturated fat in butter. Many newer margarines do not contain trans fats, and some contain a cholesterol-lowering ingredient. If you eat small servings of butter or margarine (less than one teaspoon per day) and are on a healthy, balanced diet, it really doesn't matter whether you choose butter or margarine. Go for the taste you prefer.

212 When processed is better than fresh.

In most cases, fresh fruit and vegetables are better than processed. But there is one major exception. Cooked and processed tomatoes contain lycopene—a phytochemical like beta carotene—that is utilized more readily by the body. In fact, ounce per ounce, tomato sauce, paste, or juice contains two to 10 times as much available lycopene as fresh tomatoes.

213 Go for the dark green…and red.

The darkest-colored fruits and vegetables have more vitamins and minerals than their lighter-colored cousins. And the darker plant pigments themselves may protect against chronic disease because they contain high levels of antioxidants. Choose kale, spinach, or romaine over iceberg lettuce, yams over white potatoes, red grapes over green.

214 Check package labels for reformulation.

You may have decided to buy a certain packaged food based on its attractive nutritional numbers in a magazine or newspaper article.

But don't stop there—do a little more research. Especially if you cut out that article a while back "for future reference," as many of us do, check the package label against the article. Ingredients may have been added or subtracted, and any or all of those enticing numbers may have changed.

215 Low-carbohydrate doesn't always mean "good for you."

Read package labels carefully. Many times a food or snack will contain a small quantity of carbohydrates—but will be high in calories because it is high in fat. And somewhere on the label in microscopic print will appear the words: "Not a low-calorie food."

Similarly, a food will claim low calories, carbohydrates, and fat—but for an unrealistically tiny portion. If you suspect this mendacious tactic, double the calories and other numbers for a realistic portion size, and then see if it *still* looks like a dieter's dream.

216 Peel appeal.

Don't peel apples or pears before you eat them. The peels contain most of the fiber, nutrients, and antioxidants that are so vital to our health. Instead, wash the fruits first to get rid of any pesticides. Apples and pears are two fruits that appear on the Environmental Working Group's "Dirty Dozen" list for pesticide residue (EWG.org), so it's best to buy them organic.

217 Spy a delicious way to keep the doctor away.

The variety of apples you eat makes a big difference, with Red Delicious and Northern Spy topping the list of highest antioxidant levels. In a Canadian study of eight apple varieties, antioxidant levels were five times higher in the skin of Red Delicious than in its flesh. and three times higher in the skin of Northern Spy than in its flesh.

New varieties to try: Gravenstein, Honeycrisp, Liberty, Pink Lady, RubyFrost, and SnapDragon. Gold Rush will keep in the refrigerator for nine months.

218 Delicious fiber foods.

Tasty fiber is *not* an oxymoron. We don't have to eat stuff that tastes like saw-dust or drink gritty supplements to get the 20 to 35 grams of fiber per day that doctors recommend.

Here are some tempting choices:

	GRAMS OF FIBER PER SERVING
Legumes	
Pinto beans (½ cup)	10
Red kidney beans (½ cup)	8
Black beans (½ cup)	7
Grains	
Buckwheat groats (kasha) (½ cup)	10
Barley (½ cup)	7
Fruits	
Raspberries (six ounces)	8
Blackberries (six ounces)	7
Apple	6
Mango	4
Vegetables	
Avocado (½ cup)	9
Acorn squash (½ cup)	9
Artichoke	6
Sweet potato	5

The numbers really tail off from here. If you don't see your favorite food, it wasn't in the top three or four in its category.

219 Tiny treats head off diet disasters.

Sometimes you get the urge for a snack or candy that can contain several hundred calories and lots of carbohydrates and fat. Try a sugar-free, fat-free treat that offers a tasty flavor kick instead. For example, instead of a chocolate peanut butter cup, or even a serving of peanut butter, try a little minty treat such as Tic Tacs or any sugar-free mint that contains less than 10 calories in a two-piece serving. The package is clearly labeled "Not a low-calorie food." But the flavor of these tiny treats is so intense that it may satisfy your urge.

220 Sugar alcohols can cause gastrointestinal woes.

Sugar alcohols are used as sweeteners in "sugar-free" foods. Look for ingredi-ents that end in "itol" to identify them. Mannitol, sorbitol, and xylitol are the most common, but erithritol, lactilol, and maltilol are also used. If you are sensitive to sugar alcohols, as little as 10 to 15 grams—the amount in one serving of sweetened food—can trigger severe gastrointestinal pain and problems.

221 Make supermarket design work for you.

Most supermarkets share a similar layout, with refrigerated cases along the outside walls. These contain dairy, meat, fish, and frozen foods. Produce is usually located on an unrefrigerated outside wall, and packaged foods and nonfood items are placed on shelves in the middle of the store.

People who want to eat healthfully should choose most of their foods from the fresh or frozen areas. Shopping from these outside aisles also saves lots of time.

222 Never shop on an empty stomach.

When you are hungry, you are much more likely to buy food on impulse, and that usually means snack foods. Grab some cubes of lowfat cheese, some slices of turkey breast, or a piece of fruit as you head out the door, and you won't be tempted. Your food bills will be smaller, too.

223 Outsmart mindless munching.

If the package of pretzels that was supposed to last all week is gone in an afternoon, you may be a mindless muncher.

You can break this habit, which will help you lose weight.

Keep a food diary and write down all your snacks for one week. Spot your patterns. If you find yourself snacking in the late afternoon, for example, substitute lowfat cheese or a handful of walnuts or almonds. Take a short break, get out into the fresh air and walk around the block, or phone a friend.

224 Banish your guilt feelings.

The binge-and-guilt pattern is very self-destructive and usually leads to more feelings of guilt and more bingeing in order to feel better.

You'll do better—and lose more weight—if you substitute deep breathing for emotional eating. Deep breathing lowers levels of the stress hormone cortisol, so you're not tempted to soothe yourself with food. Deep breathing also raises levels of the "feel-good" hormone serotonin twice as long as any comfort food like pasta.

225 Some cereals aren't "berry" good for you.

Freeze-dried berries or fruit in the new cereals sound like a good thing, but convenience is about all they offer. They contain only a tablespoon of the freeze-dried fruit per box but, thanks to USDA verbiage, it can qualify as a "serving" because this tiny amount will be "reconstituted" with the milk that you add to your cereal.

The fruit versions also contain substantially more sugar and less protein and fiber. For example, Cheerios contain 20 grams of carbohydrate, but only 1 gram of sugar and 3 grams each of protein and fiber. But Apple Cinnamon Cheerios contain 24 grams of carbohydrate, 10 grams of sugar, 2 grams of protein, and 2 grams of fiber. Very Berry Cheerios contain 22 grams of carbohydrate, 9 grams of sugar, 2 grams of protein, and 2 grams of fiber. Probably the worst offender is Blueberry Morning, with a whopping 45 grams of carbohydrate, 17 grams of sugar, 3.5 grams of protein, and 2.3 grams of fiber.

You'll do much better putting the fruit in yourself. Top high-fiber bran cereal with a sliced apple and a sprinkle of cinnamon, or fresh or freeze-dried berries.

226 Go wild…rice.

Switching from white or brown rice to wild rice is a healthy move—and with good reason. Wild rice isn't a member of the rice family, it's an aquatic grass. It has a similar calorie count, but twice the protein and fiber, almost four times as much potassium, six times the iron, seven times the vitamin B-1, 24 times the vitamin B-2, and almost four times the vitamin B-3 as white rice.

Although wild rice looks expensive, it quadruples when cooked, so an 8-ounce package makes six to eight servings.

227 Keep your liquids no-calorie or low-calorie.

Unfortunately, our brains don't register the calories in liquids. That's because they don't stay in our stomachs long enough for us to begin to feel full. As a result, many thoughtful nutritionists call soda "liquid candy" and criticize the supersizing of servings up from 12 ounces, with 150 calories, 44 grams of carbohydrates, and the equivalent of 10 teaspoons of sugar some years ago to the current 20 ounces, with 250 calories, 65 grams of carbohydrates, and the equivalent of 17 teaspoons of sugar. The 50-ounce 7-Eleven Double Gulp is the prizewinner, with over 600 calories, over 200 grams of carbohydrates, and the equivalent of 52 teaspoons of sugar.

Diet soda is an obvious solution to this sugary problem, but flavored seltzer, with 0 calories and 0 grams of carbohydrate per serving may be a healthier alternative, as it contains no artificial coloring.

228 Don't buy food for guests until the day they're expected.

We've all made this mistake: We buy special food because we're expecting company and we've been trained to be hospitable. That means offering them food.

But these treats are tempting, and often we succumb and start snacking on them. To avoid temptation and weight gain and sabotaging your blood glucose, delay buying goodies for your guests until the last minute.

229 Pray off your weight.

Prayer is able to move mountains, and recent research shows that it can also move mountains of flesh.

Supporters claim that prayer or meditation soothes your brain's stress center so that it does not produce cortisol, the hormone that makes your heart race and increases your appetite for fatty food. Instead, your brain produces serotonin, the hormone that makes you feel happy, relaxed, and not hungry—especially for high-calorie carbohydrates. As a result, you'll lose weight more easily because you're not eating out of anxiety and stress.

Advocates of this plan urge you to pray or meditate before each meal and whenever your resolve starts wobbling, and to write your prayer, which can be customized for boredom or emotional eaters, on index cards that you can put on the refrigerator, in your wallet, or on your desk.

230 Choose safer snacks.

Have veggies dipped in salsa or hummus, not chips dunked in dip. (Veggies also take longer to eat.)

Turkey has less than half the calories and only a fraction of the fat of prime rib.

No surprise here: Fresh fruits and berries are more healthful than buffalo wings. Even pretzels are.

231 Go for single servings.

Savvy consumers can be blindsided by choosing the "giant economy size" of a treat because it has the lowest cost per serving. But this is not a good deal for dieters.

Buy the more expensive single serving of a snack to avoid pigging out. This way you won't be able to overeat.

232 Buffets can torpedo your diet...

People love variety, and that's the problem with buffets. "All you can eat"—and so many choices!

Scientists actually discovered that people consumed more calories when they were given three different *colors* of pasta, even though they were otherwise identical. When the scientists repeated the experiment with three different *shapes* of pasta, the results were the same. Their subjects ate more again.

Here's the solution: Take tiny portions of the most interesting-looking foods. Taste them, and then go back to the buffet only once for the two or three dishes that you liked best.

233 ...And so can drinking.

Drinking affects your weight in two major ways. Not only does it add calories and carbohydrates to your diet, but it also lowers your inhibitions and resolve not to overeat.

Do some damage control. Don't drink on an empty stomach. Nurse your drinks. Drink wine spritzers—heavy on the club soda, please—or alcoholic drinks that use lots of diet soda or tonic.

234 An appetizing strategy.

Order two appetizers instead of a main course. You'll actually eat less.

235 Join a support group.

The success of support groups like Weight Watchers and Overeaters Anonymous is well known. Some newer support groups, which may be even more useful, are specifically for people with diabetes. (Being an admittedly impatient New Yorker, I'd try a support group for no more than three meetings, then decide whether it's worth continuing to go.)

236 Know where dangerous trans fats lurk.

Trans fats (partially hydrogenated oils) have been linked to type 2 diabetes, coronary disease, and strokes.

As I said in Tip 171, the FDA has ruled that trans fats are not "generally recognized as safe" and set a three-year time limit (June 18, 2018) for their removal from all processed foods.

Meanwhile, knowing which types of foods are most likely to contain trans fats will help you avoid buying and eating them. *Among the culprits...*

Cakes
Cookies
Crackers
Doughnuts

Foods fried in (partially) hydrogenated fats—e.g., chicken, fish, potatoes
Margarines (some)
Pies
Vegetable shortenings

237 Avoid "diet" bars and shakes.

"Diet" bars and shakes are loaded with many kinds of sugar. Some of the bars contain as many as 30 to 35 grams of carbohydrates and an entire thesaurus of sugars.

Some bars contain as many as eight different kinds of sugar: Corn syrup, high-fructose corn syrup, sugar, brown sugar, maltodextrin, dextrose, honey, and high-maltose corn syrup.

The first seven ingredients of one diet shake are fructose (sugar), maltodextrin (sugar), cocoa, dextrose (sugar), soy protein, sugar, and cornstarch, which is metabolized rapidly into sugar.

238 Become a "sweets snob."

Make a bargain with yourself—and keep it!—to pass up trash-food candy and carbs and indulge only in gourmet goodies. You can quash a craving better with one chocolatier's truffle than with a mass-produced mostly-corn-syrup candy bar from the vending machine or a whole bag of bargain chocolate-chip cookies—and you'd come out ahead calorie- and sugar-wise. Training yourself to savor one high-class treat is smarter and better for your body and your self-esteem.

239 Put a face on your slips and choices.

The sneakiest part of diabetes is that you don't pay for today's binge until sometime down the road instead of paying the price immediately. Sit down and examine some real equivalents. Today's candy bar could take one day off your vision in 10 years. The sour cream, butter, and carbs in today's loaded baked potato could be worth two toes in three birthdays. Having a clear picture of what an indulgence costs really helps you say no without feeling martyred because you know what you're trading for with your choice.

240 Defat before digging in.

Cut the fat from your soups and stews, and you'll cut calories without sacrificing the taste. Just toss three or four ice cubes into the pot, or one into each bowl. Wait one minute, then scoop out the ice and the congealed fat sticking to it, and discard.

If you are cooking today for tomorrow's dinner, refrigerating the dish for at least four hours will solidify all the fat, which you can then remove easily.

241 Experiment with marinades.

Brushing meat or fish with marinade can change its flavor completely. (For me, it's probably the only way I'll eat chicken breast three times a week.)

Start with a liquid—vegetable juice (lemon, tomato, or vegetable other than carrot) or flavored vinegar (balsamic, sherry, red or white wine), and add herbs and spices (dried onions, shallots, or garlic), a mix of peppers, chives, rosemary, basil, or a premixed blend, like McCormick.

Take notes so you'll remember your successes.

242 Recognize that sugar is an addiction.

Many recent research studies have linked sugar consumption to major medical problems, not the least of which is the present pandemic of obesity in the industrialized world. In the United States alone, our rate is now more than 150 pounds of sugar per year for every man, woman, and child—almost one-half pound every single day.

Possibly the best book on the subject was published back in 1975: *Sugar Blues* by William Dufty, which connects refined sugar to a laundry list of diseases in striking detail and proves his case through the centuries, with many historical documents.

The best way to determine whether sugar is an addiction for you is to examine your own eating patterns. If you find that those tempting white crystals are as addictive as narcotics and are turning you into a "sugar junkie," go cold turkey as though sugar were a hard drug. Your diabetes will improve dramatically!

243 Brown sugar and honey aren't much better.

Sure, brown sugar is less refined than white, and honey is a natural food that fearless cavemen fought bees and bears to feast on. However, practically speaking, while honey contains antioxidants and many B vitamins, it cannot be considered a significant source of them. About the only benefit of honey is that there are hundreds of varieties, and that the rich subtlety of its taste may limit the size of your serving.

244 Don't let the pounds creep up.

It's a sad fact of life that the average adult gains two pounds a year just because of slowing metabolism. Doesn't sound like much, but it translates to 20 pounds per decade.

Keep an eye on the scale and try to be more active—even if it's just a short walk after dinner.

It's easier to lose five pounds than 50!

245 It's great to grate.

Add lots of powerful flavor with no or minimal calories by grating small quantities of savory foods on top of your dishes.

Try hard cheeses, nuts, nutmeg, orange, lemon, and lime rinds.

246 Shape controls consumption.

We oughtta be smarter and not influenced by optical illusions. Nevertheless, people pour more liquid into—and then drink more out of—short, wide glasses than tall, narrow glasses holding the same number of ounces.

Choose the long, skinny glass every time!

247 Restaurant savvy VI: Be proud you're particular.

There's no need to flinch over asking waitpersons what's in a dish, or if the cream be left out, or the number of ounces in a portion. If they don't know—and really, they should—they can ask the kitchen. We live in a world of lactose-intolerant people, gluten-sensitive people, Atkins and Zone Diet adherents, and all sorts of other eating problems and programs. As long as you are polite, reasonable, and specific in your request, don't shy away from asking for some special adjustment. And if your waitperson is gracious and compliant, please tip a little extra!

248 Restaurant savvy VII: Don't let a menu blow your fuses.

Too many restaurant menus have too many choices—and too many temptations. Sometimes reading florid descriptions of dishes is all it takes to kick up a craving, so don't. Rather than let the option lead you, see what you're in the mood for and choose without even opening the menu. That way, you will order exactly what you want—or something very much like it—without being seduced by what the restaurant wants to sell you.

249 Restaurant savvy VIII: Don't reinvent the wheel.

The key to eating food prepared by others is knowing what you're eating, and how much you're consuming. Many chain restaurants regulate their recipes and portion sizes, and have that information available on request; choose those establishments. Check the menu for nutrition information, or ask your server whether pamphlets with those details are available.

250 Restaurant savvy IX: "Supersize" is a four-letter word.

Extra-hearty portions mean extra calories and extra trouble on a platter. If you suspect that a serving will be heftier than it should be, don't even let it hit your plate. Ask the kitchen to serve you only *half* of their customary portion, and to wrap the rest "to go." Clever you—you'll treat your taste buds to what they really wanted, feel no deprivation because you've finished everything on your plate, and even carry away tomorrow's lunch or dinner!

251 Restaurant savvy X: Buffet success.

Buffets are only for the truly disciplined. The good news is that you can sample a bit of this and a taste of that, and have a great time grazing. The horrible news is that the entire array is laid out to tempt you, with heavy-mayonnaise-and-pasta dishes right next to the celery sticks. Even worse, there's no portion control; you have to estimate how much you're consuming. If you're part of a group determined to gorge at a smorgasbord, you can go along—just don't even look at the layout. Specify your needs, and ask a trusted friend to fill a plate for you. Just one.

252 Restaurant savvy XI: Never eat what you don't recognize.

Stay with food you recognize and know how to calculate: a small baked white or sweet potato, green vegetables, grilled skinless chicken breast or fish, steaks listed by weight, etc. Avoid dishes that combine several foods in unknown amounts because you can't guess well. Something baked, grilled, broiled, or poached is always preferable to something fried, sauteed, or breaded. And if your entree comes covered with gravy or sauce, send it back and ask for the same thing, but "naked."

253 The devil's in the density.

Suppose you knew that a three- or four-ounce portion of a food contained 1,000 calories. (Many fast foods do.) Wouldn't eating it frequently make you put on weight?

A high number of calories per ounce of food is called "energy (calorie) density." Unfortunately, the appetite-control center in your brain signals feelings of fullness after a certain *weight* or *volume* of food has been eaten, rather than a certain number of calories.

And that's why you'll never put on weight gorging on celery sticks!

254 No catch in this rye.

Rye bread causes a smaller blood-glucose rise than eating wheat or corn bread. Researchers from Finland tested types of rye bread, containing different amounts of fiber, but concluded that the lower blood-glucose rise was not due to the fiber content, which varied. Experiments showed that rye starch metabolized more slowly than did wheat starch.

255 Be skeptical of the Dietary Guidelines Advisory Committee.

We'd all like to believe that the members of the Dietary Guidelines Advisory Committee (DGAC) a group that reviews scientific papers on health and nutrition and advises the U.S. Department of Health and Human Services and the U.S. Department of Agriculture on revisions to Americans' dietary guidelines, are impartial and unbiased.

We'd be very naive. According to the watchdog group Center for Science in the Public Interest, some DGAC members have received substantial funding from the sugar, dairy, and other food-industry groups and drug companies. Purportedly members have conducted research funded by the Sugar Association. Another has worked closely with the American Council on Science & Health, an industry group that minimizes virtually every food-related health concern, including trans fats.

Bottom line: Find trustworthy, independent verification of any DGAC report, or simply ignore it. You can guess who's buttering *their* bread!

256 Defeat diet saboteurs I: "I made your favorite dish."

Loving partners, mothers, grandmothers, siblings, aunts, and children can be the most powerful diet saboteurs because they know how to push our buttons and make us feel guilty by refusing them.

Here are two simple strategies to defeat them: Say, "Darling, I'll just have a forkful—or spoonful," and stick to your guns, or "Darling, you'll have to phone my doctor for permission. Here's the phone number."

257 Defeat diet saboteurs II: Friends and coworkers.

Sometimes these folks are well-meaning; sometimes they have hidden agendas, like the friends who don't want you to succeed at losing weight because they need to lose weight, too.

Again, here are two simple strategies for outwitting them: Play with the food on your plate, but don't eat it or eat only a tiny bit. Or say simply, "I'd love to try this, but my allergies would make me break out in hives." You'll be off the hook!

258 The real seafood diet.

You know the old joke: "I'm on a seafood diet. When I see food, I eat it."

But a seafood diet is extremely low in calories and can help you lose weight. A six-ounce serving of fish or shellfish contains less than 250 calories, with virtually no fat. In contrast, a six-ounce serving of lean broiled beef can contain 450 to 500 calories, with 20 to 30 grams of fat. Pork has even more calories and is even higher in fat. Lamb, veal, and chicken are better, but are still much higher than seafood.

259 The lure of lobster.

Lobster is the best "diet bargain." A seven-ounce portion of lobster meat (equal to a one-pound lobster) contains less than 200 calories and 2 grams of fat, and provides a whopping 35 grams of protein.

Eating a steamed or broiled lobster is time-consuming, so you'll definitely have time to feel full before you overeat. It is "fiddle food" par excellence!

Note: Most Northeastern cities have stores where you can buy live lobsters wholesale. Culls—lobsters that have lost one claw in a fight—are special bargains!

260 The sweet addiction.

Eating sweets can trigger the desire to eat more and more of them. Curb your craving by delaying these delights until *after* you eat a meal or snack that contains protein. You'll be less likely to go overboard.

261 Chart your weight loss.

A column of numbers charting your weekly weight may be OK, but you'll become more motivated by seeing a downward-sloping line on a chart. Post it on your refrigerator, where it will act as a continuing inspiration.

262 Natural weight versus idealized weight.

Your idealized weight is a product of insurance-company statistics. It is formulaic and represents hundreds of thousands of people. For many of us, it has little connection to reality.

Instead, strive for your "natural weight"—what you weighed when you were in your twenties, if you were somewhat active. Chances are that you will never have the shape of a *Vogue* or *GQ* model, but they have to starve themselves because the camera makes them appear 20 pounds heavier. Ditch any unrealistic weight-loss expectations, but stay focused on achievable goals.

263 Calcium may boost weight loss.

According to analytical research out of Creighton University (Nebraska) published in the *Journal of the American College of Nutrition,* adding two full servings of healthful calcium (such as milk and yogurt) to a diet of varied dairy intake could lower the risk of becoming overweight by as much as 70%. Other studies have shown that low-calcium diets make the body release *calcitriol,* a hormone that not only increases absorption of calcium in the intestines (so that you get the most calcium possible from food), but also causes your fat cells to make and store more fat. Of course, if you're eating healthy calcium (watch out for yogurts and ice creams with added sugar), you're not eating junk!

264 Make peace with food.

Food is not your friend. Food is not your enemy. Food is simply food—nourishment—and sometimes it's delicious.

It's time to "decriminalize" food and to savor the best of it. Slowly.

265 Orange you smart I: An orange a day.

Oranges may do more for your health than the proverbial daily apple. Multiple studies have shown that *limonin* (the substance contained in citrus fruits that provides the bitter tang in the tasty sweet) fights cancer cells. It also boosts immunity against nasty infections. So limonin plus vitamin C makes oranges a nutrition powerhouse!

Plus: Oranges possess some of the highest level of antioxidants of all fruits, with more than 170 different phytochemicals, including more than 60 bioflavonoids having anti-inflammatory and antitumor properties.

266 Orange you smart II: Eat more orange foods.

Orange-colored foods are extremely high in antioxidants, phytochemicals, and bioflavonoids, but are not always inexpensive or easy to find, especially in the winter. Look for dried apricots (but don't eat too many at one time), sweet potatoes, winter squash and, when you can find them, orange sweet peppers. (Eat carrots, too, if they don't raise your blood glucose too much.)

267 Get nutty II.

Nuts are an excellent source of protein, minerals like manganese and zinc, and B vitamins and folate. Walnuts, almonds, and pecans are especially rich in these nutrients, although the calorie counts and nutritional content vary slightly.

Note: Peanuts belong to other botanical classes. Peanuts are legumes, like beans and peas, but are eaten like other nuts and are closer to nuts than to beans in their nutritional composition.

268 Healthy dessert.

I owe this quick, easy treat to my late grandmother, who always served it to guests with or without dinner. Just stuff dried apricots or pitted prunes with walnut halves and serve them in a pretty crystal dish. (My grandmother rolled these morsels in sugar, but we know better, and they are tastier without all the additional sweetening.) *One caution:* Because pieces of fruit or nuts look so small, they may seem harmless, but in fact they're high in carbohydrates—so limit yourself to just a few pieces a day.

269 Snack on sunflower seeds.

Sunflower seeds are high in fiber, vitamin E, calcium, protein, and polyunsaturated fat, and low in carbohydrates and sugars. Grow the tall, beautiful flowers in your yard or on your terrace, and pull out the ripe seeds, or buy the unsalted variety in a health-food store. Sunflower seeds—and the equally tasty pumpkin seeds—have been harvested and used by Native Americans for thousands of years, even ground into flour.

Additional snacking bonus: Cracking the seeds in your teeth slows down your rate of consumption.

270 Flavored coffee for dessert.

Save hundreds of calories by choosing a flavored coffee for dessert. Opt for gourmet varieties like hazelnut, chocolate, raspberry, mocha, or vanilla. All of them have so few calories that you can even top your coffee with one teaspoon of ice cream and stay under 50 calories.

271 Gourmet teas for health.

Green, black, and herbal teas are all rich in flavonoids, which provide cardiovascular benefits. Recent research indicates that frequent tea drinking may affect the endothelium (the lining of the heart) favorably, which can protect your heart from cardiovascular disease.

272 Bet on berries.

All fresh berries are marvelous nutritional bargains. One delicious, filling cup of berries will "cost" you anywhere from 45 calories and 10 grams of carbohy-

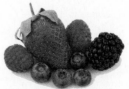

Photo: Wavebreakmedia Ltd.

78

drate for strawberries…and up to only 82 calories and 20 grams of carbohydrate for blueberries. Raspberries and blackberries fall in between. In addition, berries are loaded with antioxidants and phytochemicals.

Frozen whole berries offer essentially the same nutrients as fresh berries, but have a mushy texture so they work better as ingredients in a dish, rather than being eaten alone. Just make sure that they have been frozen without sugar!

273 An ounce of prevention is worth points on your glucose meter.

Many people with diabetes use those "I need something right now" moments to justify grabbing something they shouldn't. Plan ahead to outwit those occasions. Keep cut-up pieces of fruit in plastic containers in the refrigerator, or in plastic bags in your handbag or briefcase. Carry one-ounce portions of peanuts, almonds, or walnuts in your purse or pocket. Make those "grab something" moments into "grab something *smart*" moments and do yourself a favor instead of an injury.

274 Snack well on popcorn.

Popcorn is a healthy nibble if you make it yourself—and it's much better tasting, too. Most "manufactured" popcorn was packaged months ago and may contain strange fats.

Packaged microwave popcorn is fresher, but not necessarily better nutritionally.

But you can make popcorn from scratch right in your microwave; the hot air will make it pop without any oil. When you make popcorn this way, it's a dieter's dream. Three tablespoons of unpopped kernels will produce six cups popped, with 110 calories, 27 grams of carbohydrate, only one gram of sugar, four grams of protein, and a hefty seven grams of fiber. (That's less than 20 calories per cup, and *very* satisfying!)

Buying popcorn in the kernel is a bargain hunter's dream, too. You can usually find a two-pound bag, which will produce 23 servings, for around $3.

275 Put parsley on everything.

Parsley is a dieter's friend. An entire cup contains only 22 calories, with 4 grams of carbohydrate, 1 gram of sugar, 2 grams of fiber, and 2 grams of protein. It provides 101% of the Recommended Daily Allowance of vitamin A, 133% of the RDA of vitamin C, and is a very good source of calcium, copper, folate, iron, and potassium.

So make parsley part of your cuisine. Put it into soups, stews, and salads, use it as a garnish, and nibble it all by itself.

276 Weight loss reduces arthritis risk.

If you are 10 to 20 pounds overweight, losing as little as 10 of those excess pounds will reduce your risk of developing osteoarthritis by 50%, according to John Klippel, MD, former president and CEO of the Arthritis Foundation.

If you are more than 20 pounds overweight, you will need to lose more than 10 pounds to reduce your osteoarthritis risk significantly. It's definitely worth it!

277 Try the "white-out" diet.

Many people with diabetes can achieve substantial weight loss with a "white-out" diet: Eliminating white bread, flour, rice, sugar (in its many forms), potatoes, and cornstarch. No surprise—all of these foods have high glycemic indexes and make most diabetics' blood glucose rise very quickly.

278 Substitute carob for cocoa.

Health-food fans support the strategy; chocoholics think it's heresy.

The answer probably lies somewhere in between. Compared with baking cocoa, carob powder—sometimes called "carob flour"—is only slightly lower in calories, but contains more than twice as many grams of carbohydrate, half of which are sugar. Carob contains three times as much fiber, but no protein or iron, and cocoa contains both. Carob contains no fat, but cocoa contains very little.

Before sugar substitutes were available, the natural sweetness of carob was an advantage because its users did not have to add sugar the way cocoa users did. And the sugar added all the calories and carbohydrates.

Now the playing field is more level. Chocolate lovers can choose based on their taste preferences.

279 Cocktail party strategy.

Ya gotta walk around with a drink in your hand, right? But that means you can't hold an hors d'oeuvre in that hand!

Here are some look-alike drinks that will keep your calories and alcohol consumption down...

Virgin Mary instead of a Bloody Mary

Club soda or tonic with a wedge of lime instead of gin (or vodka) and tonic

Or substitute a wine spritzer for a glass of wine

280 Resist nibbling with rest.

Dieters who get enough sleep find it easier to stay with their weight-loss programs. According to recent research, dieters who classified themselves as "well-rested" snacked less and lost more weight than those who said they weren't getting enough sleep.

Try a catnap instead of cookies to restore your energy!

281 Color your world.

You already know that you should be consuming lots of antioxidants to keep healthy and prevent damage by free radicals. Colorful vegetables and fruits have the antioxidants that you need...and, don't forget, you eat with your eyes! Pretty food makes a healthy meal a sumptuous delight.

Lunch on colors: Instead of just boring celery sticks with your midday meal, peel and cut up sweet potatoes, carrots and beets (yes, they're yummy raw... but they tend to color everything they touch)...wash up bright string beans, broccoli flowerettes, slices of yellow, orange or red peppers (see also Tip 266) and munch away the beautiful array.

Pair dishes with colorful sides: Instead of a plate full of brown items such as chicken and rice, liven up your plate with deeply colored fruits and vegetables that add variety and important phytonutrients (components of fruits and vegetables that are thought to promote health) to your diet.

282 Low-carbohydrate diet? Consult your doctor and lower your insulin.

It's not because your doctor will try to persuade you to choose a "more balanced" diet. In fact, many doctors have lost weight on Atkins and other low-carbohydrate diets and are among their most vocal supporters.

But if your insulin and other hypoglycemic drugs are not lowered, you can go into sudden shock and die. Case in point, told to me by a prominent Manhattan internist who is a happy Atkins dieter...

One of his patients, a diabetic in his 30s, went on the Atkins diet without having his insulin changed—and died quite suddenly from hypoglycemic shock.

So—to reiterate—if you are lowering your carbohydrate intake, you MUST have your insulin and other hypoglycemic drugs lowered.

283 Don't drink too much water at one time.

Drinking too much water at one time is dangerous. It's very tempting to drink a quart of water or more within a few minutes to make sure you get your daily quota, but drinking too much water too quickly leads to a dangerous dilution of the salt and other electrolytes in your blood, causing "water intoxication" that may require hospitalization. Older people are especially vulnerable to this serious problem.

Instead, unless you have been exercising or it is very hot, drink only one or two cups of water at a time, and sip slowly. Let your thirst be your guide.

284 Betcha *can* eat just one.

Many calorie, carbohydrate, and fat counts for snacks are based on a serving of more than one piece. A serving of Hershey Kisses, for example, is based on seven pieces and contains 160 calories, 19 grams of carbohydrate, and 9 grams of fat.

Try eating just one, letting it dissolve in your mouth slowly and pleasurably. Then you're talking about a very manageable 23 calories, and about 2.7 grams of carbohydrate and 1.3 grams of fat.

285 Try six little meals a day.

You may be able to lose more weight on six little meals a day. Same number of daily calories, if you're counting them, but spread out more.

Such a weight-loss program works for many dieters—not just people with diabetes—for two major reasons: They are less tempted to overeat because they are eating so often, and the frequent meals keep their metabolic furnace stoked up so they burn more calories.

286 Buy the family size, then divide.

Supermarkets often put cuts of meat and fish in "family-sized" packages, which can save you over $2 per pound.

Take advantage of these bargains, then cut and wrap individual portions and freeze them.

287 Try brochettes.

Brochettes are a tasty, quick-fix dish. You've probably tasted this Middle Eastern lamb dish, which comes in many varieties. It's low in calories and fat, high in protein and vitamins.

Thread cubes of meat, chicken, or fish on a skewer, alternating with chunks of onion, pepper, tomato, or other vegetables. Broil in the oven or rotisserie, or on the barbecue.

288 Experiment with stir-fries.

Stir-fry recipes are another tasty way to increase the vegetable content of your dinners. Try stir-fries with asparagus, snow peas, spinach, Chinese cabbage (bok choy), broccoli, hot or sweet peppers, all varieties of mushrooms, onions, or scallions.

289 Drop the two-hour lunch.

Two-hour lunches are too tempting. Too many opportunities to eat too much food, or just sit around, which slows your metabolism.

Instead, take only an hour for lunch, then go shopping or take a walk with your lunch companion.

290 Avoid overly restrictive diets.

Sure, they may work for a week or two, but they may also create a feeling of deprivation. When it gets too strong, your diet may backfire and cause you to go on an eating jag. It's much smarter to start your diet by making a list of 10 or 12 foods that you absolutely will not eat. Anything else is OK as long as you control your portions.

291 Don't quit smoking and start dieting at the same time.

Taking on two deprivations at once is almost a recipe for failure. Quit smoking first. Not only will it start you on the way to a healthier future, but you will also redeem your taste buds. When you begin your diet a month or two later, you will really savor your food and find it easier to lose weight.

292 Spend your fast-food allowance on kitchen gadgets.

Whether it's a pepper or salt mill, an apple corer, a cherry pitter, a lemon zester, or mushroom slicer, it's an inexpensive investment in making food look and taste better quickly and easily. Doesn't that make more sense than spending your money on fast-food meals or coffee breaks?

293 Picture perfect.

Make the old adage, "One picture is worth a thousand words," reinforce your weight-loss plan.

Put some photos on your refrigerator for continuing inspiration. Choose a photo of yourself when you were in high school or college, or a newlywed, and weighed much less. You could attach your face to a movie star's or athlete's body—preferably in a bathing suit. Write the caption "MY GOAL" on it and keep on focusing on that goal—especially every time you go to the refrigerator.

Note: If negative stimuli inspire you more, put a photo of yourself at your present weight on the fridge.

294 Supplement a microwave meal with a green salad and fresh fruit.

Microwave meals can be lifesavers after a long day at work. Make them healthier by adding a green salad and fresh fruit or berries for more vitamins, fiber, and antioxidants.

And toss the starch, noodles, or rice in the meal.

295 Stay away from cereal bars.

Cereal bars are a poor nutritional bargain. They are promoted as a quick, portable breakfast. But many of them are loaded with all kinds of sugars, and some still contain trans fats. (What really irks me is seeing "high-fructose corn syrup" first or second on the list of ingredients, followed immediately by "corn syrup." Now, really!)

Some cereal bars are somewhat more nutritious, but you'll have to read the labels carefully; 250 calories is a heavy "price" to pay.

296 Put your pet on a diet, too.

Many dogs and cats are now as overweight or obese as their loving owners. As a result, many of them have become diabetic, with all the cardiovascular risk that their owners face.

The best thing you can do to increase your pet's life—and your own—is to put both of you on a diet. Limit snacks and increase exercise. Check first with your vet.

297 Bean benefits.

Beans have a lot going for them. Not only are they an excellent source of low-fat protein and fiber, but they also provide substantial iron and folic acid.

I like the versatility of beans—especially red kidney beans, white beans (cannellini), and pinto beans. With a blender or food processor, you can make a soup or dip very quickly. Or make a bean salad for a nourishing hot-weather dinner.

Recent research suggests that high-fiber beans can increase weight loss by 66%, according to a study published in *Nutrition Reviews*. Says Michigan State University nutrition professor Maurice Bennink, PhD, "Getting at least 30 grams of fiber a day (½ cup of kidney beans contains 23 grams) can significantly speed dieting success—even without exercise or other lifestyle changes."

298 Chocolate lover? The darker, the better for you.

The most healthful chocolate you can eat is the darkest. Search for chocolate labeled a minimum of 70% cocoa solids, which has a high concentration of heart-healthy phytochemicals and iron, and very little sugar and carbohydrates. Higher concentrations of 72%, 85%, and 90% cocoa are even more healthy.

You can sometimes find pound-plus bars of this gourmet chocolate at specialty supermarkets like Trader Joe's for as little as $5, a true chocolate lover's bargain.

299 Yo-yo dieting increases health risks.

Losing weight and regaining it all, then losing weight again and gaining it back has harmful consequences. This yo-yo dieting, which is more likely to occur with women than men, can increase the risk of cardiovascular disease, already the number-one killer of women in the United States. Yo-yo dieting can also lower the levels of "good" HDL cholesterol and raise triglycerides, an independent risk factor for heart disease in women.

300 Don't try to be "the greatest loser."

In "After 'The Biggest Loser,' Their Bodies Fought to Regain Weight," a brilliant May 2, 2016, article, *New York Times* medical author Gina Kolata followed the contestants of Season 8 of NBC's reality TV show. She discovered, by interviewing metabolism experts, that six years later, the contestants' metabolisms had become even slower. Worse, they had to consume far fewer calories than normal to keep from gaining back *more* weight. As Kolata pointed out, "Dieters are at the mercy of their own bodies, which muster hormones and an altered metabolic rate to pull them back to their old weights, whether that is hundreds of pounds more or that extra 10 or 15 that many people are trying to keep off."

So what's the answer? Probably to be "The Most Permanent Loser," keeping those 10 or 15 pounds off year after year. Crash dieting really doesn't work.

301 Try the triple-mirror test.

Sometime during the winter holidays, you may need encouragement to stay with your weight-loss plan. (Admittedly, all those fabulous parties don't help.)

Strengthen your resolve by going to an upscale department store that has a cruisewear department and try on some bathing suits in a triple-mirrored dressing room. Look at your body from all angles. What you see—and what you'd like to see in a few months—may inspire you to stay on the straight and narrow and not abandon your diet.

302 Give yourself a hand.

Maybe you're tired of weighing your food—I know I am!—or there are situations where you can't. *Estimate your portion size by comparing it with your hand…*

One thumb = 1 tablespoon, or 1 ounce of cheese

One palm (or a deck of cards) = 3 ounces of meat
One fist = 8 ounces of liquid, or 1 cup of solid food

303 Pumpkins: Not just for pie.

Pumpkins are a wonderful winter food because they are an excellent source of vitamin A (it's their bright orange color!) and such minerals as potassium and phosphorus.

All this nutrition comes at a low caloric cost. One cup of pumpkin cubes contains only 30 calories, with 8 grams of carbohydrate and only a trace of fat. If you love pumpkin pie, put the cubes in a blender or food processor, then simmer them with powdered ginger and nutmeg and a sugar substitute for a sweet treat. Or simmer the pumpkin cubes with dried sage to get the taste of pumpkin ravioli without the dough, calories, and carbohydrates.

Tip: Pumpkins usually go on sale November 1, the day after Halloween, and often right after Thanksgiving.

304 Vim and vinegar...

Vinegars contribute a variety of interesting flavors while adding zero calories. This category has changed a lot in the past 10 years as old supermarket standbys like red, white, and cider vinegars have been joined by balsamic, malt, sherry, tarragon, and raspberry. Seasoned rice vinegar contains sugar, so be sure to choose the plain variety.

Try different varieties on salads, vegetables, meat, poultry, and fish. Raspberry vinegar is especially tasty on melons, berries, and fruit.

305 ...And other condiments and sauces.

Here, too, you can add a lot of flavor without adding significant calories or carbohydrates. An assortment of condiments can make the blandness of chicken breasts disappear. Drizzle them on cooked vegetables to disguise their taste—maybe you'll eat more of them. Tabasco anyone?

306 "Natural" doesn't mean "healthful."

Packaged-food manufacturers love to make their products sound as if they're good for you. The labeling "naturally sweetened" is one of the most insidious sales and marketing tools because it tempts us to buy something—most often a snack—that is nutritious and "good for us."

I've got news for you: Sugar is a natural sweetener. So is molasses, which is made from sugar cane. So is honey. And so—stretching the point just a bit—is xylitol, a sugar alcohol made from birch bark, which causes horrendous gastrointestinal problems in many people in portions as small as 10 milligrams (one-third ounce). In fact, if sawdust were sweet, it, too, could be labeled a "natural sweetener." (It comes from trees, doesn't it?) If you think I'm kidding, before the 1980s, sawdust was added to many brands of "diet bread" to increase their fiber content.

307 Neither does "organic."

According to USDA labeling, "organic" has to do with certain prohibitions in the way food is grown. Organic foods cannot be genetically engineered or modified, cannot be fertilized by sewage sludge or irradiated, and cannot be fed animal-slaughter by-products, antibiotics, or growth hormones.

Clearly, then, organic food may be the choice of food purists, "free-range" fans, opponents of agribusinesses, and chefs.

However, that said, the caloric, carbohydrate, and fat content of many packaged "organic" foods may be so high that people with diabetes should avoid them or eat them very sparingly. "Organic" doesn't mean "you don't have to read the label."

308 Sneaky labeling: "No cholesterol."

And now we come to really sneaky labeling: Packaged foods marked "no cholesterol." For too many foods, these words are misleading because, while legally true, the food never did contain cholesterol, which comes from animal sources.

For example, a package of potato chips fried in many types of vegetable oil, which is high in saturated fats that are very harmful to the cardiovascular system, could legally be labeled "no cholesterol." And so could a loaf of bread made with partially hydrogenated vegetable oil, another cardiovascular villain.

A package of frozen vegetables could also be labeled "no cholesterol." Of course, vegetables *never* contain cholesterol—unless they're packaged in butter or cream sauce.

You'll be healthier if you ignore the "no cholesterol" labeling and concentrate instead on what the food *does* contain.

309 Get the goods on granola.

Granola conjures up all sorts of warm and fuzzy feelings—kind of like yogurt, sandals, and sunshine.

But granola may not be so healthful for people with diabetes. Many varieties of granola still contain partially hydrogenated vegetable oils, 210 calories in a half-cup serving, with 36 grams of carbohydrate and only 4 grams of fiber and 6 grams of protein. (And who eats only a ½-cup, anyway?) In contrast, a ½-cup of Fiber One cereal contains only 60 calories, 25 grams of carbohydrate,

14 grams of fiber (10 grams of net carbohydrate), but, sadly, only 2 grams of protein.

310 Watch calories as well as fiber content.

Cereals can be a good source of desirable fiber; we need 30 to 40 grams of it per day. But cereals are among the most important packaged foods whose labeling you must read very carefully. Even "bran" and "fiber" cereals may contain too many calories, carbohydrates, and sugars to be good for you, and there is a great deal of variation among the hundreds of different cereals.

For example, Post Raisin Bran contains 190 calories in a one-cup serving, with 47 grams of carbohydrate, 8 grams of fiber, and 5 grams of protein. Post Bran Flakes contains 100 calories in a ¾-cup serving, with 24 grams of carbohydrate, 6 grams of fiber, and 3 grams of protein. Original Shredded Wheat, which you might think would be high in fiber, has only 80 calories per biscuit, but only 2.5 grams of fiber.

311 Make friends with your supermarket manager.

Make a point of learning your manager's first name and greeting him whenever you see him. Treating him like a person, rather than a job title, lets you find out useful information, like what will be on sale next week, and lets you ask him for favors, like ordering special foods and merchandise for you.

312 Know the dark side of supermarket design.

Have you ever wondered why the dairy case is usually in the back of the supermarket? To make you go through lots of aisles and look at lots and lots of merchandise before you can get to the quart of milk you came in for. That way, maybe you'll buy some other things as well.

Similarly, staple items are scattered all over supermarkets so that you have to visit every aisle. That's why most people find it difficult to finish the weekly shopping trip in less than 15 minutes.

Foods with high markups are usually piled attractively at the end of aisles. That's because it takes you a little longer to turn your cart around—more time for you to be tempted. Other high-markup items are placed at your eye level, or your child's.

Now that you know the secret, you can avoid a lot of that deliberately engineered temptation. Just stick to your shopping list—except maybe for just one treat and good sales on items you normally buy.

313 **You're not through when you get to the checkout counter.**

You're in the checkout line with your shopping cart. You've bought everything on your list and avoided all the temptations.

Stop! There's one more obstacle to navigate: All those tempting goodies racked up next to the cashier, often in snack-sized packages. Why do you think the store does that? Because managers know about impulse purchases.

What to do? If you absolutely, positively must, buy the smallest little goodie—just one, please. But if you can, pass those temptations on by and give yourself a hug for being a weight-loss hero.

314 **Outwit the winter weight-gain syndrome.**

Genetically, we haven't changed much from our Stone Age ancestors who ate what they could in the late fall and winter because they never knew when their next hunt would take place, or whether it would be successful.

These ancient traits survive in us as unconscious habits. Maybe it's the cold and dark affecting our psyches. We tend to eat more in the winter and to gain weight—hopefully to lose it in the spring.

Now that we recognize the psychological component of winter weight gain, how can we outwit it? Dishes that need long cooking will soothe your inner caveperson without piling on the pounds. Try experimenting with soups, stews, and casseroles. The aromas of the long, slow cooking and the warmth of your kitchen will satisfy your emotional needs and help you avoid overeating.

315 **This "ade" won't help you.**

Orangeade, lemonade, and other fruit drinks sound "natural" and "healthy." But check their labeling. According to the USDA, a fruit "ade" can contain as little as 15% fruit juice. The other 85% can be sugar and water, high-fructose corn syrup and water, or anything else. An 8-ounce serving often contains over 200 calories. Not the best choice for people with diabetes!

(And, of course, remember that as bad as fruit drinks are, drinking a lot of pure fruit juice isn't good for people with diabetes, either.)

Healthier choice: Eat a piece of fruit, drink lots of water, seltzer, or no-calorie flavored seltzer.

316 **Substitute olives for chips or pretzels.**

Try olives when you're in the mood to snack on something salty. Although olives contain fat, it's monounsaturated fat, good for cardiac health. And the average green olive contains fewer than 10 calories, so it's better nutritionally than chips, which are often cooked in partially hydrogenated vegetable oil, or even pretzels, which contain mostly flour.

Besides, while many of us have devoured an entire bag of chips or pretzels at least once in our lives, who among us has wolfed down a whole bottle of olives?

317 Pickles, too.

Those little cornichons (baby pickles) that accompany pâté in good French restaurants can be nibbled on their own when you're in a snacking mode, so they're truly a "free" food.

Other varieties of pickles are larger and contain more calories, but you're more likely to be satisfied with fewer of them. Experiment with dill, sour, half-sour, mustard—all easy to find, all tasty.

318 Pick frozen produce...

Frozen fruits and vegetables are available all year 'round in your supermarket's freezer case. Because they are flash-frozen at the peak of ripeness, except for differences in texture, they are as tasty and nutritious as fresh produce. Possibly even more so, because they have been processed more quickly before being shipped.

319 ...And frozen desserts.

While you're at the freezer case, check out the frozen desserts. You can enjoy many of them and still lose weight.

Among my favorites: No Sugar Added Fudgsicles (40 calories, 10 grams of carbohydrates), Tofutti Chocolate Fudge Treats (30 calories, 6 grams of carbohydrates), and Dole No Sugar Added, Tropicana Sugar-Free, and Welch's Sugar-Free Fruit Bars (25 calories, 6 grams of carbohydrates each).

320 "It's on sale" is not a good enough reason.

Food manufacturers and supermarket chains spend billions of dollars a year to persuade you to buy their foods. No, it's not conspiracy theory—just the facts of life. One of their most profitable merchandising tools is the weekly flyer that highlights the foods that are on sale—complete with brightly colored pictures and juicy prices.

Fight back! Become a more educated consumer. Sale prices are not a good enough reason to buy specific foods, just as they're not a good enough reason to buy other merchandise you don't need.

Bonus: When you stop buying food just because it's on sale, you save money as well as lose weight.

321 Read new food claims carefully.

Thanks to new, loosened USDA regulations, almost any food can claim almost any health benefit—regardless of any research—as long as the label uses such vague "weasel words" as "evidence supports but is not conclusive," "bone strength," or "heart health." Skip the advertising claims, read the ingredients and their percentage of the adult RDA (Recommended Daily Allowance), then judge for yourself.

322 *Really* know how sweet it is.

Food labeling is shown in grams, which doesn't help those of us who are still more comfortable with teaspoons.

Get a better idea of how sweet a packaged food is (and whether you should eat it) by using this formula: To calculate the number of teaspoons, divide the grams of carbohydrate or sugar by 4.2. Thus, a premium ice cream that contains 46 grams of carbohydrate in a half-cup serving has nearly 11 teaspoons of carbohydrate—mostly sugar—in that serving.

323 Psych yourself into vegetables I: Maybe you're a supertaster.

If you've hated vegetables since you were a kid, there's a good chance that you're a supertaster. This term is used to describe people who are extremely sensitive to bitter tastes because their tongues possess an unusually large number of taste buds.

It's not necessary to stick out your tongue and inspect it in a mirror. If you've always been a picky eater, rejected most vegetables, and asked for sauce and dressings on the side, you're most likely a supertaster.

As vegetables are so important in a healthful diet, read the tips in this section for ideas on how to make vegetables more palatable.

324 Psych yourself into vegetables II: Start with the sweet ones.

Sweet vegetables have lots of vitamins and are easy to get used to. To make them even tastier, add grated orange rind, cinnamon, or ginger to carrots, sweet potatoes, or pumpkins, allspice to zucchini, and mint to green peas.

325 Psych yourself into vegetables III: Seek perfection.

We've all experienced vegetables that weren't served at peak ripeness—woody asparagus, flabby tomatoes. No wonder they tasted terrible!

Other than growing your own and picking them just before dinner, your best bet is to buy produce in peak season at farmers' markets or greenmarkets. Spend some time chatting with the farmers and with fellow customers. Learn the characteristics of the most desirable vegetables and also how to store and prepare them. Admittedly, the best, freshest vegetables will be more expensive than the usual supermarket offerings, but you'll find them worth it.

326 Psych yourself into vegetables IV: Ban bitterness with blanching.

Blanching vegetables before cooking them makes them much less bitter. This technique works especially well on cancer-fighting cruciferous vegetables: Broccoli, Brussels sprouts, cauliflower, broccoli rabe. Steam or boil them for about a minute, then remove them and plunge them into cold water. This stops strong flavors from developing.

Tip: Use blanching to remove skins from tomatoes.

327 Psych yourself into vegetables V: Babies may be better.

Baby vegetables usually have milder flavor; the flavor gets stronger as they mature. And baby vegetables are more tender, so they require less cooking time. You can find them at farmers' markets or specialty grocers. Some baby vegetables are even available frozen.

328 Psych yourself into vegetables VI: Drizzle with butter or oil.

A teaspoon of butter or herb-infused olive oil won't wreck your diet and may persuade you to eat more vegetables because fat makes all food taste better. Even truffle-flavored olive oil can be an affordable treat one teaspoon at a time!

329 Psych yourself into vegetables VII: Sprinkle with cheese.

We're not talking about your grandmother's heavy, fattening cheese sauce here! A teaspoon of crumbled blue cheese or grated Parmesan sprinkled over your vegetables can transform their taste.

330 Psych yourself into vegetables VIII: Sneak veggies into other dishes.

Making an omelet? Throw in some cubed onions and green or red peppers. Top with sliced mushrooms. A meat loaf? Blend in a cup of grated onion or zucchini. Muffins? Some grated carrots or zucchini. Soups or stews? Let your imagination run wild. All of these contribute sneakily to the number of servings of vegetables to eat every day.

331 Psych yourself into vegetables IX: Add a little spice.

Have you always disliked spinach? Sprinkle it with nutmeg. Cabbage? Cook it with caraway seeds, mustard, or both. Kidney beans are the main ingredients in chili, so adding chili powder and cumin is a natural. Tomatoes are enhanced by many herbs and spices—basil, garlic, oregano, peppers of all types, and rosemary, for starters. Experiment!

332 A low-fat diet may increase diabetes risk.

A low-fat diet often leads to a greater consumption of carbohydrates—especially from refined flour—according to a Harvard School of Public Health study of more than 42,000 men aged 40 to 75. The study, which was published in *Annals of Internal Medicine* in February 2002, suggested that such a high-carbohydrate diet could be worse for health than a high-fat diet, as it increased the risk of diabetes.

Smarter choice: Whole-grain products and healthful fats, like olive oil. If you think this sounds like the "Mediterranean diet," you're right!

333 Customize your weight-loss plan.

A session with a nutritionist may be just what you need to jump-start your weight-loss plan. A good nutritionist will take a detailed medical and eating history and will ask pointed questions in order to design a weight-loss program that you will be more likely to stay on.

334 Focus on what you *can* eat.

The typical supermarket sells more than 30,000 items, of which more than two-thirds are food. That's 20,000 choices. Even if you can't eat half of these, that still leaves you 10,000 foods you can choose from. You'll be more successful if you focus on what you *can* eat, not what you can't.

335 Learn to like salmon.

I don't mean lox, the mainstay of so many weekend brunches. We really can't eat four ounces of the fish, and smoking this tasty delicacy removes many of its nutritional benefits.

Especially compared with lean beef, lean pork, or turkey breast, it makes sense to add salmon to your diet. Here are the statistics per four-ounce serving…Beef contains 212 calories, 8 grams of fat, and 34 grams of protein. Pork contains 163 calories, 4 grams of fat, and 30 grams of protein. Turkey breast has 153 calories, only 0.8 grams of fat, and 34 grams of protein. Salmon contains 120 calories, 2 grams of fat, and 26 grams of protein. If you compare calories with protein in each choice, salmon is clearly an excellent nutritional bet!

336 Recognize that being overweight runs in families.

Whether it's genetic or environmental—sharing the same menu, going back for second helpings—being overweight runs in families.

Make weight loss run in your family instead. Get your family on a weight-loss program. Create your own in-house support system. You'll all benefit!

337 Visit the ethnic-foods shelves of your supermarket.

The ethnic-foods shelves of your supermarket can surprise you with food choices you never thought of, in many combinations and sizes. Most supermarkets devote lots of space to Hispanic and Asian cuisine. Browse here for interesting vegetable combinations, sauces, and seasonings.

338 Track your snack attacks.

If you're having trouble losing weight, you may have selective amnesia about your visits to the refrigerator and pantry.

Here's an easy way to check: Start each day by putting a Post-It adhesive note and a pen or pencil on the refrigerator. Every time you open the fridge or go to the pantry, note the time and what you ate. When you go to bed, stick the Post-It in a notebook and date it. At the end of a week, you'll have an excellent record of when you're snacking, what and how much, and how you need to change your routine to break this habit.

339 Set up little goals and big ones.

People who lose weight successfully choose both short-term and long-term goals. Losing 50 pounds is intimidating, but not if you start with a smaller, short-term goal of losing 10 pounds in the first month, then five to 10 pounds per month over the next four or five months. Setting and achieving goals one step at a time creates a feeling of accomplishment so that you're more likely to continue. Remember the old adage: "The journey of a thousand miles begins with a single step."

340 Gotta binge? I: Try this catechism.

The urge to binge hits us all at one time or another. Here are some ways to deal with it:

Ask yourself: "On a scale of 1 to 5, with 5 being the maximum, how strong is this urge?" Be honest!

Ask yourself: "Can I wait 10 minutes?" Set a kitchen timer and wait for it to ring.

Ask yourself: "If I knew that this binge would damage my eyes/kidneys/feet, would I still do it?" You probably wouldn't!

341 Gotta binge? II: Keep a "safe-snack" shelf.

Having a "safe-snack" area that you have set aside in your refrigerator will minimize the effects of bingeing. Keep it well stocked at all times so that you won't feel deprived.

What you put there depends on your food preferences. *Here are some suggestions...*

Canned water-pack chicken breast or tuna
Low-fat cheeses
Hard-boiled eggs
Cut-up vegetables
Cherry tomatoes
Mushrooms
Tomato or vegetable juice
Sugar-free Jell-O

342 Binge substitutes I: Sweet.

So you crave something sweet. You have lots of sugar-free, no- and low-calorie choices. Among them: No- calorie soda and flavored seltzer, sugar-free Popsicles and fruit-juice pops, Fudgsicles, and Jell-O.

If it's chocolate you desire, try my recipes for guilt-free chocolate milk (Tip 103), or rum, cognac, or Grand Marnier truffles (Tip 105).

Or if you lust after apple pie, try my two quick apple pie substitute recipes (Tips 195 and 196).

343 Binge substitutes II: Creamy.

So you crave something creamy. First, choose whether you want something sweet or something rich, like a high-fat cheese.

For something sweet, try my five Guilt-Free Cheesecake recipes at the end of this chapter.

For something rich, like Boursin, a garlic-herb cream-style cheese, make your own low-fat yogurt cheese (Tip 199). Blend in garlic powder or slivered garlic, chives, parsley, and your favorite herbs after the whey has drained out of the yogurt.

344 Binge substitutes III: Salty.

Often it's the salt we really crave, rather than the pretzels or potato chips. If that's the case, skip the onion and sour-cream potato chips. Instead, try mixing onion salt into some low-fat yogurt to achieve the same flavor.

For the crunch of pretzels with a little extra taste, grab a small handful of bacon-flavored soy bits. Or snack on a small dish of olives or pickles.

345 Fast food? Check online first.

Fast food can still be an option if you do your homework first, rather than ordering impulsively without knowing the calorie, carbohydrate, fat, and protein content of your choice. Among the fast-food chains that post the nutritional content of their dishes online are Burger King, Hardee's, McDonald's, Ruby Tuesday, Subway, TGI Fridays, and Wendy's. There are hundreds more at DietFacts.com.

346 Snack on soy.

Soy snacks can be an excellent substitute for potato chips. Not only are they lower in calories and fat, but they also contain soy protein, which offers cardiovascular benefits by lowering cholesterol. There are lots of flavor choices, including barbecue, cheddar, nacho, ranch, and salt vinegar. For the best selection, try a large supermarket or health-food store.

347 Good eating habits make you healthier than the average person.

The silver lining in our diabetic cloud is that developing good eating habits and controlling our weight will make us healthier than the average person.

According to the Centers for Disease Control, more than 60% of American adults are overweight, and many of them are obese. According to the World Health Organization, obesity is a worldwide epidemic. And obesity is linked to many other diseases: Cardiovascular, hypertension, stroke, arthritis, and joint problems for starters.

Eating sensibly and carefully can put us ahead of the average American, who doesn't. For firsthand empirical evidence, just look at the contents of the shopping carts on your next trip to the supermarket, and at the weight of the customers pushing them.

348 Orange you smart III.

Eating an orange? Eat the pith—the white fiber—too. That's where most of the fiber is, plus a lot of the antioxidants.

349 Cocoa lowers cancer risk.

Diabetes raises cancer risk. Now there's a tasty way to lower it...

In a study published in *Journal of Agricultural and Food Chemistry* in 2003, Cornell University researchers reported that a cup of hot cocoa (pure cocoa powder and water) contains twice the quantity of phenolic phytochemicals—powerful cancer-fighting antioxidants—found in a glass of red wine, three times the quantity found in a cup of green tea, and five times the quantity found in a cup of black tea. The antioxidants protect against cancer by ridding the body of damaging free radicals.

Note: Previous research suggests that adding milk to the cocoa could block its antioxidant action.

350 Variety is the key to your weight-loss success.

Let's face it: Most diets fail because they are too restrictive and boring. Eventually dieters cry: "Let me outta here!" But if you can choose from among hundreds of healthful foods prepared in many different ways, you actually have *thousands* of possibilities, even if you're a picky eater.

When you realize the vast number of options, you are much more likely to stick with your diet—or even rotate among weight-loss programs after a few months or so—and keep on losing weight!

351 Steam—don't microwave—your veggies.

Produce loses as much as 97% of its flavonoids, a type of potent antioxidant, when it is microwaved, according to a research study from the Department of Food Technology, a major research center in Murcia, Spain. Microwaving destroyed the highest percentage of flavonoids, followed by conventional boiling.

Steaming preserved almost all the flavonoids, so steam your veggies or eat them raw for maximum nutrition.

352 Five-pound weight swings are meaningless.

Don't panic if your weight fluctuates from day to day. Weight swings of five pounds have no significance because they can be caused by water retention and many other factors. In fact, these five-pound weight swings can occur if you weigh yourself three or four times a day, as many obsessive dieters do.

You can get a better sense of whether you're losing weight by weighing yourself only once a week.

353 Don't hide from your scale.

Not weighing yourself at all is just as self-destructive as weighing yourself after every time you go to the bathroom. Not weighing yourself for months makes you the king or queen of denial. Psychologists call this hiding from the scale "avoidance behavior": You don't want to be confronted by the cold, hard numbers showing how much you've overeaten.

Instead, use your scale as a helpful tool to keep you focused on your weight-loss program and all the advantages your weight loss will give you.

354 Dine to slow music.

Listening to sweet, stately music while you eat slows you down. You relax, take more time at the table, but actually eat less while enjoying it more.

Here's the science behind it: We speed up unconsciously to fast music, and dawdle to slow music. Eating more slowly gives our brains time to signal our stomachs that we are full.

Try chamber music, opera or ballet music, symphonic works by the great classical masters from your own library, or classical FM stations.

355 Form a lunch bunch.

If you have congenial coworkers who enjoy tasting new foods, try this:

For a group of five, choose one person to bring lunch for everyone on Monday, another person on Tuesday, and so on. Discuss food preferences so that everyone will be able to eat something every day, and nobody will feel unhappy.

This lunch club will save you lots of money and time. If you go for a walk after lunch, you'll burn some extra calories, too.

356 Know that all protein metabolizes into carbohydrates.

It has to, so your body can use it. This means that you have to be careful with a super-high-protein diet. That 16-ounce steak will probably raise your blood glucose the next day, even though it's wonderful as a once-a-week treat.

357 What kind of eater are you? I: All or nothing.

In her inspirational book *Plan D*, Sherri Shepherd, actress and former cohost of TV's *The View*, confesses to a "love affair" with Pinkberry frozen yogurt that escalated into an outright addiction. When she realized that she couldn't just downsize—it had to be an all-or-nothing decision—she vowed never to eat frozen yogurt again.

358 What kind of eater are you? II: Happy eating the same foods.

If you need to lose weight and have to get to work in a hurry, you can really enjoy the same food for breakfast every day—and similar foods for lunch and dinner. For example, you might try the same easy, delicious breakfast every day: Fresh berries or fruit, low-fat cottage cheese with cinnamon (which makes insulin work better), a small handful of walnuts, a one-ounce chocolate walnut cookie (fewer calories and grams of carbohydrate than most cereal portions), and a large cup of coffee with a little 2% milk. No sweetener—that's what the cookie is for.

Take a break on the weekend with a cheese omelet and a couple of strips of turkey bacon.

I inject a short- and long-acting insulin before breakfast and dinner, so I eat a smaller lunch: Low-fat cheese, turkey breast, one thin slice of whole-grain flaxseed bread, and three-quarters of an ounce of 85% or 90% cocoa chocolate.

Dinner has larger portions of meat or fish, raw vegetables or a salad, and a little ice cream.

359 What kind of eater are you III: Eat fast? Try a "square meal."

My late friend, science-fiction author Isaac Asimov, virtually inhaled his meals, a habit carried over from childhood, so that he'd have more time for reading. If you share this bad habit, try this eating game I learned decades ago in Girl Scout camp:

You must lift every fork and spoon in 90-degree movements: up, out, and down to pick up your food, then up and into your mouth, out and down to your plate. See how much you've slowed down?

If your kids gobble their meals, this is a great family game!

In the spirit and intent of *1,137 Secrets for Living Well with Diabetes*, I end this chapter with several recipes for "guilt-free" cheesecakes.

It's rich, creamy, and not too sweet. Cheesecake is a favorite dessert that many dieters hate to deny themselves. But a portion of plain Cheescake Factory cheesecake contains a whopping 710 calories, 49 grams of carbohydrate, and 49 grams of fat. Fruit-flavored cheesecakes are even more fattening.

OK, I admit that the recipes that follow have no crusts. But that's where the calories and carbohydrates lurk and—let's face it—the appeal of cheesecake is not its crust.

What you'll find here are recipes ranging from as little as 91 calories to a maximum of 190 calories per serving, with five to 17 grams of carbohydrate, two to seven grams of fat, and as much as 22 grams of protein per serving.

Enjoy them!

360 Guilt-Free Cheesecake I: Coeur a la Creme

(Serves two)

> 1 cup low-fat cottage cheese
> 2 ounces Neufchatel cheese, slightly softened
> Pinch of salt
> Several envelopes of sugar substitute, to taste
> 1 cup fresh strawberries, raspberries, or blueberries

Thoroughly blend all ingredients except berries in a bowl. Refrigerate.

About 15 minutes before serving, shape the cheese into a heart, place on a pretty serving platter, and surround with berries.

Approximately 190 calories, 12 grams of carbohydrate (mostly from the berries), 7 grams of fat, and 19 grams of protein per serving.

361 Guilt-Free Cheesecake II: Mascarpone with Apricots or Peaches
(Serves four to six)

Mascarpone, named after the eponymous Italian cream cheese, is a more sybaritic version of the French Coeur a la Creme.

4 ounces whipped low-fat cottage cheese
4 ounces Neufchatel cheese, slightly softened
¼ cup plain low-fat yogurt
Several envelopes sugar substitute, to taste
2 tablespoons Grand Marnier, cognac, or light rum
Fresh apricot or peach halves

Combine all ingredients except fruit in a large bowl. Beat until well blended. Mound in a cone on a pretty serving dish and surround with the apricot or peach halves.

Spoon a little of the cheese mixture into the fruit half and eat.

Based on four servings, approximately 136 calories, 6 grams of carbohydrate, 7 grams of fat, and 9 grams of protein per serving. Three apricots per serving add 51 calories and 12 grams of carbohydrate; one peach adds 37 calories and 10 grams of carbohydrate.

362 Guilt-Free Cheesecake III: Lemon Cheesecake
(Serves four)

2 large eggs
2 cups low-fat cottage cheese
2 teaspoons vanilla extract
2 teaspoons lemon extract
2 tablespoons fresh lemon juice
2 tablespoons nonfat milk powder
1 envelope sugar substitute
2 egg whites
Pinch cream of tartar
Butter-flavored vegetable spray
Preheat oven to 350 degrees.

Mix all ingredients except egg whites and cream of tartar in a large bowl. Beat egg whites and cream of tartar until stiff peaks form, then fold into other ingredients.

Pour into springform pan greased with butter-flavored vegetable spray. Bake for 30 to 35 minutes. Cool. Refrigerate overnight. Before serving, garnish with grated lemon peel, if desired.

Approximately 151 calories, 5 grams carbohydrate, 4 grams fat, 22 grams protein per serving.

363 Guilt-Free Cheesecake IV: Strawberry Cheesecake

(Serves two)

2 teaspoons sugar-free strawberry Jell-O
1 tablespoon hot water
1 cup strawberries, reserving several of the prettiest for garnish
⅔ cup low-fat cottage cheese
1 large egg white
1 teaspoon almond extract

Dissolve Jell-O in hot water. Blend strawberries and cottage cheese in blender and add Jell-O mixture.

Beat egg white until stiff. Add almond extract to berry mixture. Fold in egg white. Chill in a serving bowl until set and garnish with remaining strawberries.

Variation: Substitute sugar-free raspberry Jell-O, raspberries, and vanilla extract.

Approximately 91 calories, 7 grams carbohydrate, less than 1 gram fat, and 4 grams protein for either version.

364 Guilt-free Cheesecake V: Cherry Cheesecake

(Serves eight)

3 large eggs, separated
1 pound farmer cheese or pot cheese
4 envelopes sugar substitute
½ teaspoon vanilla extract
¼ teaspoon cinnamon

Cherry Glaze

1 large can water-packed cherries, pitted
1 tablespoon cornstarch
1 envelope sugar substitute
Few drops red food coloring (optional)

If you can't find either farmer or pot cheese, you'll need to start this recipe a day early. Put 1½ pounds of cottage cheese in a very fine sieve placed over a bowl, and put it in the refrigerator. The whey (liquid) will drain into the bowl, leaving you with the pot cheese.

Preheat oven to 325 degrees.

Place egg yolks and other ingredients in blender. Blend at low speed until smooth.

Meanwhile, beat egg whites until peaks form.

Place cheese mixture into a bowl and gently fold in egg whites.

Pour mixture into a springform pan greased with butter-flavored spray. Bake 15 minutes.

Turn oven up to 450 degrees and bake five minutes more. Remove cake from oven and prepare Cherry Glaze.

Drain cherries, reserving liquid. Add cornstarch and mix until well blended. Heat mixture over medium flame until it starts simmering and is slightly thickened. Remove from flame, add sugar substitute and food coloring, and mix thoroughly.

Place the cherries on top of the cheesecake and spoon the glaze over them. Refrigerate the cake in the springform pan for several hours to overnight before unmolding and serving.

The glaze firms as it chills.

Approximately 92 calories, 9 grams carbohydrate, 2 grams fat, and 9 grams protein per serving.

CHAPTER 3

Working with Your Doctors and Other Health-Care Professionals

365 Newly diagnosed? How you got here.

Maybe diabetes runs in your family, but you may not have had any symptoms—no excessive thirst, no weight loss. And then one day your lab tests show that you're spilling sugar into your urine, meaning that you have so much glucose in your blood that it has overflowed into your urine.

Now that you know, managing your diabetes is up to you. You may be able to reverse it with a lot of self-discipline and hard work, or at least to manage it successfully. This book's tips will help you!

366 "Can the doctor please call me before my appointment?"

Save this tip for your most serious concerns, and for when your appointment is at least a week away. Most doctors are happy to solve little problems over the phone, before they become bigger ones.

367 Know the difference between "urgent" and "emergency."

"Urgent" and "emergency" are terms that medical staff recognize and respond to; they're learned in triage classes. "Urgent" is serious, but a one-hour delay is not critical. "Emergency" is a "10" on a 10-point scale, like bleeding that won't stop. Call 911, head for the emergency room and, when you arrive, ask the medical staff to contact your doctor.

368 Be a "good" patient.

"Good" by our standards, *not* theirs. This is not the same as taking your doctor's every word as gospel.

Bring a list of questions to every appointment. Keep a log of your blood-glucose readings and bring that, too, and bring your blood-glucose meter for your doctor to download and print out. Show that you are very motivated

103

about preventing serious complications; some diabetic patients aren't. (I think they're in denial.)

Let your doctor know that you won't pester him/her, but if you phone, it means that you're in *serious* trouble and need a quick call back or appointment. Suggest this as a "treatment contract."

Ideally—especially if you are insulin-dependent—your doctor will let you fax or e-mail weekly logs and then call you if there are unusual readings or patterns, or if your medication needs adjusting. As a result, you probably will have fewer extreme high and low blood-glucose readings. Just search "Diabetes" in the app store.

369 Know your doctor's treatment style.

When it comes to drugs and treatments, some doctors are traditional and conservative ("Let's stay with this old drug—it has a long safety record") and some prefer new ones ("This drug has lots of new features"). Both viewpoints are legitimate and reasonable; the question is which is closer to yours.

370 Key: Your medical history and this test.

Every competent doctor will ask you to provide a complete family medical history. But in the case of diabetes, both type 1 and type 2 can manifest in the same family. Many doctors will not necessarily order a C-peptide test, which measures how much insulin your body produces, and then will determine whether you have type 1 or type 2 diabetes. Even though the treatments for type 1 and type 2 can be similar, and thus doctors may feel that this information is not essential, request it as part of your treatment so that you know for sure, from the beginning, which condition you have.

371 Don't accept bad medical care.

An endocrinologist I saw—once—broke off our appointment to see a drug-company salesman. As I waited for him to return, my blood glucose tanked and I started getting hypoglycemic symptoms.

When he returned and I told him what was happening, he started chewing me out.

Not only did I never see him again, but I told my family doctor and also wrote to the medical group's president. That endocrinologist is not working at the medical group anymore.

372 Testing, testing.

You should have these lab tests performed at least once a year. If your doctor doesn't order them, ask why.

●**CBC (Complete Blood Count)**—This test measures the number of red and white blood cells, whether there are any abnormalities in the number and types of white blood cells (eosinophils, basophils, neutrophils, monocytes, lymphocytes), immature ("stab") cells, and hemoglobin levels, which diagnose anemia.

●**Urine microalbumin**—This test checks the presence of the protein albumin and determines how well your kidneys are functioning.

●**Creatinine, BUN (Blood, Urea, Nitrogen)**—This is another test of how well your kidneys are functioning and preventing the buildup of toxins.

●**Lipid profile**—This test checks the levels of fats in your blood, which can be a precursor of heart attack and stroke.

●**Liver profile**—Because the liver is the major cleansing organ of the body, this test measures liver function, which can be affected by toxins—especially from drugs you are taking.

These tests should be done every three months…

●**Fasting blood glucose**—This test checks whether your fasting blood-glucose levels are too high, too low, or within acceptable range, and tells your doctor whether your medication needs to be adjusted.

●**Glycohemoglobin A1C**—Like Santa Claus coming to town, this test tells your doctor how "good" (good control) or "bad" (poor control) your blood glucose has been for the past three months, with an emphasis on the last month. There's no way to "cheat" on this test.

373 Share information with your doctors.

You have more time to read about new research and treatment for diabetes than your family doctor, who has to spread reading time over many medical topics, or even your endocrinologist, who has to read about thyroid, parathyroid, and adrenal problems, too.

Web sites for *The New England Journal of Medicine* and *The Lancet* are especially good sources. So are search engines and even the Tuesday "Science Times" section of *The New York Times* and the "Trends and Innovations" column of *IBD Weekly*.

Your doctors will appreciate your help and will likely give you better care.

374 Other specialists you should see.

Get referrals from your family doctor or endocrinologist if you need to, but see these specialists…

Cardiologist—Every six months or more often if you're taking a heart medication

Ophthalmologist—Every six months to find glaucoma, retinopathy, and other diabetic eye diseases at their earliest stages.

Podiatrist—As needed.

375 Cite a "higher authority."

Unfortunately, many family doctors and nurses are very ignorant about diabetes.

Here are some horror stories from fellow diabetics…

"I had a general practitioner tell me I was obsessive-compulsive before I was rushed to the hospital with a blood-glucose reading over 900!"

"A doctor told me to take insulin when my blood glucose was low. I had sugar pills ripped out of my hands while on the verge of passing out from hypoglycemia."

"I said a hypoglycemic reaction was coming on. I was asked to make it wait."

To educate these "medical experts" tactfully while protecting your health and sanity, cite a "higher authority." *For example*: "Doctor, did you know that the American Diabetes Association/Joslin Diabetes Center says that diabetics should have juice/sugar and water/regular soda when their blood glucose is low—not insulin?"

I hope that the ADA and Joslin won't mind!

376 Ask your doctor to check your blood pressure at every visit.

If your blood pressure is high at the beginning of the examination—the infamous "white-coat syndrome"—ask to have it checked at the end, too. Many patients who test high at the beginning because they're nervous or worried relax toward the end of the examination, so the reading is more accurate. Testing your blood pressure in both arms is a valuable diagnostic tool.

Diabetics are susceptible to many kinds of circulatory problems, so your doctor should keep a record of all your blood pressure readings.

377 Check your blood pressure frequently, too.

You really don't need your own blood pressure monitor unless you suffer from high blood pressure. (Many diabetic patients do.)

Most pharmacies have removed their blood pressure testing stations to create more profitable selling space, so I suggest buying a blood pressure monitor ($40 to $50) and check your blood pressure twice a day, at roughly the same time of day. Most monitors will store 50 to 100 readings, so bring your monitor to your cardiology appointments for downloading and diagnosis.

378 Get your flu shot as early as possible.

You can't afford to overlook this crucial annual ritual. People with diabetes are six times as likely to be hospitalized if they develop influenza as people without diabetes. This is a risk you can't afford to take. Other immunizations you may need are discussed in Chapter 1, Tips 35–38.

379 Before gastric bypass surgery, ask your doctor about alternatives.

Many doctors will prescribe gastric-bypass surgery for their patients who are extremely overweight or obese. Overweight is defined as 10% to 20% higher than the normal weight (the precise definition depends on which longevity expectation chart you use, frame size, muscle mass, and doctor's evaluation). As a general rule, if you think you're overweight, you probably are. Obese is defined as 20% higher than normal weight for men, 25% higher for women. Morbid (life-threatening) obesity is defined as being more than 100 pounds overweight.

If your doctor recommends gastric-bypass surgery and your medical insurance will pay for it, ask your doctor about alternatives, which are both less risky and far less expensive. Gastric-bypass surgery can cost from $15,000 to more than $35,000. In contrast, the weight-loss programs at Duke University cost only about 15% to 20% of that amount.

Gastric-bypass surgery gained more support in May 2016, with guidelines recommending weight-loss surgery as a more routine treatment option for type 2 diabetes, even for some mildly obese patients. These recommendations were endorsed by the American Diabetes Association, the International Diabetes Federation and 43 other health groups, and was published in *Diabetes Care*.

Although it may be easier to get your insurance plan to cover this surgery, it still should be considered a last resort, after you have tried losing weight for six to 12 months. (Try the tips in Chapter 2, "Weight Loss and Nutrition.") Even losing as little as two pounds a week will result in your losing 100 pounds in one year!

Let's face it: Gastric-bypass surgery is often major abdominal surgery. Even laparoscopic surgery is serious. Preparing for surgery involves several weeks of a modified diet, then fasting and drinking lots of water—slow sips, please—plus the usual presurgical exams, lab tests, and chest X rays.

The Mayo Clinic points out that you'll have to remain in the hospital for three to five days after surgery to check your healing and make sure that there are no problems.

The surgery itself poses both short-term and long-term risks, starting with the general anesthesia of surgery. Short-term risks include excessive bleeding, infection, blood clots, lung or breathing problems, leaks in your gastrointestinal system, and sometimes even death.

Long-term risks include bowel obstruction, dumping syndrome (diarrhea, nausea, vomiting), gallstones, hernias, hypoglycemia and malnutrition (because your stomach is now a tiny fraction of its original size and your small intestine is now so much shorter), stomach perforation, ulcers, vomiting, and even death.

Your postsurgical diet will be limited, too. You'll start with a liquid diet, then progress to pureed foods, and then—after about eight weeks—to chopped or diced food. You will still have to avoid spicy foods and foods with texture, although you may be able to return to some of them after three to four months.

Carbonated and alcoholic beverages will be forbidden for a very long time—possibly forever.

And remember: Gastric-bypass surgery is permanent! You may never be able to enjoy a festive meal again!

380 Nonsurgical alternatives.

In May 2017, the program at Duke University cost about $2,820 for one week, $5,175 for two weeks, $6,930 for three weeks, and $7,965 for four weeks, but seasonal discounts bring these rates down. There is also an additional per night charge for your room.

Joslin's Do-It (Diabetes Outpatient Intensive Treatment) lasts only four days, but is truly intensive, starting at approximately 7:00 a.m. and running past dinner. The program costs about $6,000 as of May 2017, plus your room at a nearby motel.

Insurance companies should be delighted to pay all your medical expenses because they are so much lower than the costs of the gastric-bypass surgery. Even more important, in most cases you will be better off learning successful new behaviors to help you lose weight and improve your health than undergoing the surgery and enduring the long-term side effects.

381 Don't be like Judy Garland.

Remember how Judy Garland's handlers gave her "uppers" so she could wake up and work and "downers" so she could rest at night...and then "uppers" again the next morning? If you're taking more than one prescription medicine, be sure to read all the fine print on the medication printout from your pharmacy.

In another multiple-drug story, a woman who was shocked when her legs started retaining fluid for the first time in her life discovered that edema (swelling) was a side effect of one of her glucose-control medications. She was also taking a diuretic to reduce her fluid retention.

Especially if you have an endocrinologist or more than one doctor treating you, take all your prescriptions to your primary-care provider for review. Make sure that your doctors aren't prescribing at cross-purposes.

382 On Medicare? You can still find a good doctor.

Many doctors limit the number of Medicare patients they accept because reimbursement payments are slow, but these strategies may work for you...

• **Mention the name of the person who referred you.** The doctor may accept you as a patient to avoid alienating the colleague or patient who referred you.

• **State that you are looking for a permanent doctor.** Doctors prefer regular patients to acute-care patients.

• **Tell the doctor if your Medicare plan is fee-for-service rather than managed care.** Reimbursement payments are higher, so the doctor will be more likely to take you on as a patient.

• **Even if you are turned down once, try again**—especially early in the year. After reviewing their finances at the end of the year, many doctors decide to accept new patients.

383 Make your doctor's staff part of your team.

Your doctor's employees are gatekeepers. They control access to your doctor. They can facilitate or roadblock your appointments and do you lots of small favors if they like you.

Case in point: A friend was able to get a flu shot immediately, rather than having to make an appointment for a separate visit several weeks later. My friend got special treatment because several months ago she asked the nurse, "Are you having a bad day? You look tired."

Treat your doctor's staff with TLC. Remember their names and little bits of personal information. Are they married? Do they have children? Pets? Are they planning a vacation? Bring them a small Christmas or Chanukah present. You'll be glad you did when you need that emergency or add-on appointment.

384 Get what you need from your insurance company.

Are you having problems getting enough supplies to test your blood glucose as frequently as necessary to keep your glycohemoglobin A1C low? Is your doctor having problems getting authorization for your supplies? *Here's how to get what you need...*

• **Most private insurance plans have a case manager who can approve individual patient requests based on special needs.** Contact the case manager and explain your treatment regimen and the supplies you need that will keep you out of hospitals and emergency rooms. Ask the case manager what documentation is needed, and get the case manager that documentation.

●**Keep on pushing for what you need.** Some states are trying to pass legislation allowing insurance plans to refuse coverage for diabetic supplies. Don't let this happen!

385 Stick with one pharmacy.

When you use only one pharmacy, your pharmacist has a record of all the drugs you are taking and can alert you to any potential drug interactions or side effects. (It's also a lot more convenient.)

386 Use a pharmacy with a good computer system.

Most chain pharmacies (and many smaller ones) print out and attach very complete drug information with every prescription.

A typical printout will include instructions on using the drug, side effects, precautions (e.g., previous allergic reactions and diseases, use during pregnancy or nursing), interactions with other drugs, what to do if you have missed a dose or have overdosed accidentally, and how to store the drug (room temperature or refrigerator).

Keep these printouts handy for future reference. Do not discard them.

387 Have your pharmacist substitute smaller needles.

Always ask your pharmacist to give you the smallest gauge needle insulin syringe available. In general, your pharmacist will not substitute a shorter needle, but will substitute a *thinner* one. The smaller gauge doesn't cost more money, and you will certainly notice the difference in comfort.

388 Get copies of your medical records.

Ask every doctor's assistant or receptionist for a copy of your medical record—and make sure that you get it. Build a file that you can refer to again and again, and research whatever diagnosis and treatment that you may not understand. Use it to develop questions for your next visit to this doctor, or to other specialists. Use it to monitor your progress.

389 Time your lab tests.

Get your lab tests done two weeks before your doctor's appointment so that they'll be ready for your doctor to review before your visit.

390 That all-important blood-glucose diary.

No matter how you create it, bring at least two weeks of your blood-glucose diary to your doctor's appointment. (Three weeks' worth is more useful if you have the time.) Write down the time of each test and the result, the timing, name, and dosage of any diabetes drugs you are taking, and any unusually heavy meals or exercise. The more complete your diary is, the more your doctor will be able to advise you.

Even if your software program lists blood-glucose readings and drug dosage, it may not cover stress, exercise, exact meals, etc. Clearly, all of these influence your blood glucose.

I keep the original of this diary, print a copy for my doctor, and bring both to every appointment. That way I can write his comments on my copy and refer to it at home.

391   As you age, your doctor may relax your blood-glucose and A1C goals.

Many diabetes specialists believe that blood-glucose and A1C targets of 120 to 150 and 6.8 to 7.2 that are perfectly suitable for patients in their 40s and 50s are riskier for patients in their 70s and 80s because of the danger of hypoglycemic falls. Therefore, these doctors are suggesting blood-glucose and A1C goals of 200 and 8.0 for their older patients. These doctors believe that it would take more than 20 years for these higher targets to do any significant damage—as long as their patients keep their weight at a healthy level and eat and exercise sensibly.

392   Your Q&A notebook.

A 4" x 6" notebook can be an invaluable tool in your medical care.

For each doctor you see, keep a running list of questions and symptoms with dates. The best way to do this is to use a double-page spread with your questions on the right-hand page. Save the left-hand page for your doctor's answers to your questions.

For example, you might list…
- **Blood pressure?**
- **Result of lab tests?**
- **Adjust medications? New prescriptions?**
- **Pain in right toes—arthritis or neuropathy? Treatment?**

Keep a different double-page for each doctor, marking the top with his/her name, specialty, and appointment date. Make a duplicate copy when you have time, and tell a family member or friend where it is and to bring it if you should need a hospital or emergency room.

393   Try a "group appointment."

One of the newest trends in patient care is the "group appointment," in which several patients share long group appointments—as opposed to short, hard-to-schedule individual appointments—and have a chance to ask all the questions that they want to.

This may work especially well for people with diabetes. Talk with your doctor about the possibilities.

394 Your friendly *neighborhood* doctor...

Several times in the last 10 or 12 years (I've had diabetes for 30+), I have owed my health—and avoided a trip to the emergency room—to a doctor who was a neighbor.

Of course it's Murphy's Law that we come down with strep throat on Friday night or Saturday morning, after regular doctors' office hours. Having a friend who lives nearby who will write that all-important prescription on a weekend—so that you can fill it immediately—can be a godsend.

395 ...And your friendly *neighborhood* urgent-care facility.

When you absolutely, positively need a doctor and don't need or want an emergency room, these small medical centers are the greatest! Think of them as a first line of defense. They treat minor injuries and often have X-ray rooms and lab facilities so they can diagnose what's causing that mysterious stomachache, rash, or whatever ails you.

Personal story: In February 2016 I realized that my persistent cough had been persistent for too long, so I hustled to my urgent-care center one Saturday morning after breakfast. (*Remember*: I'm a type 1 diabetic and I didn't want to risk hypoglycemia.) I didn't have to wait long. A medical assistant listened to my heart and lungs, took my blood pressure, drew some blood, and sent me down the hall for a chest X-ray.

Then a doctor examined me and diagnosed walking pneumonia. By the time I got to my pharmacy, a powerful 10-day antibiotic was waiting for me. Five days later, I was healthy again.

396 The best time for appointments.

Do you hate to wait? Schedule doctors' appointments, for times when you're least likely to cool your heels in the waiting room.

If you hate to wait, be the first appointment in the morning, or the first one after lunch. Call before you leave for your appointment to check whether the doctor is running late.

To guarantee *your* choice of appointment, make follow-up appointments before you leave the doctor's office. Even if your next visit isn't for many months, you'll have your choice of a pretty empty calendar, *and* you won't waste time later calling for an appointment.

397 Having diabetes does not exempt you from other diseases.

Sad but true, having diabetes may actually increase the likelihood that you have other problems—cardiovascular, vision, and others. Simply getting older brings still other diseases, like arthritis.

This means multiple doctors' appointments, but look on the bright side: Being aggressive about your medical care can prevent or delay hospitalization, and can extend your life.

398 Double up your appointments.

Because more than one doctor is taking care of you, if you belong to a medical group, it's smart to double up on your appointments. For example, see one doctor at 9:00 and another at 10:30 or 11:00 on the same day. You'll save both traveling time and time off from work.

399 Two reasons to dump your doctor. Fast and furious.

(1) being put on hold for 15 minutes
(2) not having your phone call returned in 24 hours. No excuses—you are the customer, and you are important.

400 Is your doctor board certified?

Doctors who have been practicing for more than three years should be certified by a medical board in their specialty. This certification goes beyond an MD. It is more like a postgraduate degree and is granted by one of the 24 medical boards that are members of the American Board of Medical Specialties. Most boards have certification, recertification, and maintenance certification programs to keep their doctors current in the latest developments in medicine.

You can check whether your doctors have been board certified by calling toll-free (866) 275-2267, or logging on to ABMS.org, which has links to its 24 member boards.

Note: Endocrinologists are certified by the American Board of Internal Medicine.

401 You may be covered for alternative-medicine services.

Many insurance providers are now covering such alternative-medicine services as acupuncture, massage therapy/bodywork, nutritional counseling, and mind-body relaxation treatments. Depending on your policy, these services may be discounted, or you may have to make a copayment. It's worth checking!

402 Get the most accurate blood-pressure reading.

Blood pressure is important because people with diabetes are so susceptible to cardiovascular problems.

Ask your doctor to measure the pressure in both arms, not just one. Markedly lower pressure in one arm could mean that blood vessels are partially blocked on that side and need to be checked further.

403 Find a doctor who's flexible.

You'll do better with a doctor who doesn't impose a rigid one-size-fits-all mind-set on your treatment. You want, need, and deserve a doctor who will be responsive and who will tailor a treatment program to your individual situation. Someone who will keep tweaking and fine-tuning your treatment and medications until they are the best possible fit.

404 Have your doctor check your blood-glucose meter.

At least once a year, bring your blood-glucose meter, test strips, and lancet to your doctor's appointment and ask him to test your blood glucose on your meter and on the meter in his office. Very often there are significant differences in the numbers, and you will manage your diabetes better if you work with a meter that is accurate.

It's much better to test your meter against the lab's results. The doctor's meter might not be any more accurate than yours, and many doctors and nurses aren't very sophisticated about meter technology.

405 Navigating affordable health insurance.

Examine your coverage carefully every year—health insurance plans are certain to change over time. Talk to your friends, neighbors, relatives, colleagues. Remember that even if you choose a plan that turns out to be horrible, you can always choose another one next year.

406 Your annual physical: What's all this stuff?

With all the computerized information in your doctor's office, it's likely that he/she will give you a printout contact sheet showing your current medications, future appointments and tests, and a "problem list."

Here's your opportunity to check your medications and ask your doctor to delete any you are no longer taking, add any new ones, and make sure the dosages are still correct.

The problem list can really be a problem if you are a long-term patient because it can have 40 or 50 problems, many of which can go back for years and are no longer relevant. Sometimes there is even duplication. For example, my own chart lists both "osteoporosis" and "senile osteoporosis."

This can be a problem for doctors who have to navigate these long lists. Ask your doctor whether it's possible to sort out these problems into different categories—e.g., current/chronic like your diabetes, one-time events longer than five years ago, etc.

407 Know who's covering for your doctor.

It's inevitable: You have a question or a problem after your doctor's office is closed, or on the weekend. What do you do? Whom can you call?

You *must* get the name and phone number of a doctor who covers for your own doctor. You need someone with access to your records who can answer your specific questions.

Put this doctor's name and phone number right under that of your primary-care provider, or your diabetes specialist.

408 Better doctor-patient communication I: Be an individual.

With many doctors treating as many as 100 patients a week, your first job is to remind your doctor who you are, especially if you're a fairly new patient.

Make eye contact with your doctor and make sure there's a response. Then tell your doctor about what's been happening in your life since your last visit. (Your doctor should be taking notes.)

409 Better doctor-patient communication II: Opening the window.

When you discuss your blood-glucose log and food diary with your doctor, focus on these questions: "Do you see any patterns here? Has anything changed? Should I do anything differently?"

These questions open a dialogue in which new information is exchanged. For example, your insulin dosage may need to be tweaked very slightly; adding or subtracting only one unit can make a big difference in your blood-glucose control.

It goes without saying that doctors work harder for motivated patients. You want to be one of them!

410 Better doctor-patient communication III: Discuss future goals.

At every visit, ask your doctor, "What do I need to improve? Is there anything new or different I should try?" This is especially important if you have type 2 diabetes because, according to a study published in 2002 in *Southern Medical Journal*, "Internal medicine physicians have negative attitudes toward type 2 diabetes that require future educational interventions."

411 **Better doctor-patient communication IV: Get in the loop.**

Ask your doctor to e-mail you between your visits if there are important new developments in diabetes care. (My endocrinologist emailed me about the availability of CGMs—continous glucose monitors—in January 2017, making it necessary for me to rewrite Tip 11.) Medical conferences take place year-round, and many medical journals are published weekly or monthly. You want to stay current so that you can take the best care of your diabetes.

412 **Enlarge your health-care team.**

Besides your primary care doctor, cardiologist, and your ophthalmologist, get referrals to these other professionals if you have more specific problems: An endocrinologist specializing in diabetes care and a dietitian or Certified Diabetes Educator. Many medical groups and communities also offer diabetes classes and support groups.

413 **Add a physiatrist to your team.**

Physiatry (the practice of physical and rehabilitation medicine) is a fairly new specialty; it's nonsurgical orthopedics. Physiatry covers the musculoskeletal system, so it can be useful in treating many joint and muscular problems without having to resort to surgery.

My personal opinion: I would consult a physiatrist first, then an orthopedic surgeon if nonsurgical rehabilitation treatment didn't work well enough.

414 **Doctor bills: Let's make a deal.**

You can often negotiate lower fees with doctors, dentists, hospitals, and pharmacies.

Do a little homework first. Learn how much health-insurance companies and Medicare are paying for the same services. In general, managed-care companies receive a 40% discount on medical services, and doctors will often give you a similar discount.

Start by asking your doctor, "Can you help me out? Could you please bill me what Medicare or insurance companies pay you?"

CHAPTER 4

Avoiding/Surviving Hospitals and Emergency Rooms

415 Avoid trips to the emergency room.

Remember Louis Pasteur's sage words, "Fortune favors the prepared mind," and be aware that falls cause most emergency-room visits for diabetic patients. *To avoid these frightening falls...*

1. Turn on your night-light or grab your flashlight before you get out of bed when it's dark.

2. Check your blood glucose before you get out of bed, especially if you've been asleep or napping.

3. If your blood glucose is low, eat some glucose gel or tablets. Stay in bed for 10 or 20 minutes, then test again. Now it should be safe to get out of bed and move around slowly, using a cane, walker, or surrounding furniture to "cruise" for stability.

4. If you have any weakness in your hands, arms, or legs, wait a little while longer—you don't want to risk falling.

At some point, adrenaline—that marvelous fight-or-flight brain chemical—should take over, raise your blood glucose, and make your moving around safe.

If you need to get to the bathroom in the middle of the night, there's no shame in crawling on your hands and knees or scooting on your butt. (I've done both.) Anything's better than a fall and a trip to the emergency room!

416 Getting to the emergency room.

1. Call 911 or have a friend or family member call for you.

2. When EMS gets on the phone, be as detailed as you can. Make sure your door is unlocked or contact anyone with keys (who can lock your door and take your keys, wallet or purse, and your "go" bag to the hospital if you need to go).

3. Unless your condition requires transportation to the nearest hospital, you have the legal right to demand being taken to the hospital of your choice.

Best: Request the hospital that has your medical records.

4. Speak with the EMS team as much as you can. You want to convince them of your competence and coherence—especially important if you have fallen and been unconscious for several minutes.

417 In the emergency room.

Intake and evaluation start the process. Then you are assigned to a bed and a doctor. After you are examined, your doctor will discuss a preliminary diagnosis, tests, and treatment.

418 You'll have to wait for blood-test results.

If nurses or lab technicians draw your blood in the emergency room, it will take at least two or three hours to get the results. They're doing a lot of tests in addition to blood glucose. Just be patient—your diagnosis depends on this!

419 Know your blood type.

When you are in the hospital or emergency room, crucial time is wasted if your blood must be typed before you receive a transfusion. If you don't know your blood type and it's not in your records, ask your doctor to run the proper tests at your next visit, and to record your blood type in your medical records. When you donate blood to the American Red Cross, they will supply you with a card listing your type. Keep this card handy at all times.

Make sure that you know your family members' blood types and that they know yours—just in case a transfusion is called for.

420 Wear a Medical Identification Bracelet at all times…

To indicate that this is more than just jewelry, your bracelet should have the caduceus—the international medical symbol—on it, and the words "diabetic" or "insulin," and your blood type. (You can buy these at pharmacies or have them made to order. Several medical ID organizations exist online, such as Medicalert.org.)

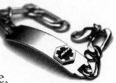

Photo: duckycards

421 …And carry a Medical ID Card in your wallet.

This card should contain information concerning allergies, blood types, treatment authorization, people to notify and other vital facts to help medical personnel diagnose your needs in a medical emergency. Printable medical ID card templates are available free online (Medids.com/free-id.php), but you might want to check out the high-tech flash drives and personalized bracelets that can contain detailed medical history—these are available through such websites as MedicalHistoryBracelet.com (210-681-3840) or AmericanMedical-ID.com (800-363-5985).

EMS and emergency-room workers are trained to search for these items if you are unconscious.

422 Keep a medication list.

Have a list of all medications that you are taking, and their dosages. If your doctor changes a medication or dosage, update your list immediately. Keep a copy of this list with you at all times so that you will have it in an emergency. *If you don't have any place to keep this list in the emergency room, then pin it to whatever you are wearing.*

You will also help your doctors—and yourself—if you include the name of your family physician and his/her phone number, as well as the name and phone number of the doctor who prescribed each medication. All this information can be contained on your Medical ID flash drive, if you choose high-tech storage (see Tip 421).

423 List your allergies.

Make a list of all your allergies (food, pollen, pets, etc.), as well as any prescription and nonprescription drugs to which you are allergic. Keep it with you or include on your Medical ID card (see Tip 421).

424 Bring your insurance cards.

Be sure to take with you any membership cards of major medical plans, HMOs, and/or Medicare, Medicaid, and AARP…and take a picture of them with your smartphone, just in case.

425 Write down all your symptoms.

As best you can, regardless of the physical and mental pain and stress you are suffering, try to write down every single symptom you are experiencing, how long you've experienced it, and how it may relate to an already-existing condition that has caused you problems before this. Unless you write down all of this, you may forget to tell the doctor the one clue that would lead to an accurate diagnosis.

426 Bring a relative or friend with you.

You may be in too much pain, or may not be coherent or conscious. Having someone with you to deal with medical personnel and hospital procedures can make you feel much less frightened and much more comfortable and can help ensure proper care.

427 Know how emergency rooms work.

Most emergency rooms operate on a two-track system. Patients who are seriously in need of immediate and possibly lifesaving treatment get to see a doctor first. This system is called triage, a term familiar to us *M*A*S*H* fans. Many hospitals also use the "fast-track system," which gets patients who need minimal attention for minor ailments and injuries in and out of the emergency room as quickly as possible.

Unless you are put on triage or on the fast-track system, chances are that you will probably have to wait for medical attention an hour or two, or even longer and much, much longer on weekend nights and holidays. Think of the gastrointestinal problems right after Thanksgiving! To make the waiting easier and less nerve-racking, take along some light reading, a few magazines, or a book of crossword puzzles to help you pass the time.

428 Make sure your doctor specifies your personal care.

Have your admitting doctor write orders stating that you have permission to test your own blood glucose, take your own medications, and order your own meals—especially if your hospitalization is not connected to your diabetes.

429 Plan for autologous transfusion.

Is elective surgery in your future? Then plan for autologous (your own blood) transfusion in case you need blood.

This is how it works: First, ask your surgeon whether your surgery might even remotely require a transfusion, and how many units of blood you might need. Then ask your surgeon what the guidelines are for your donating blood for your own use.

In general, you will have to go to your hospital's blood bank every two weeks to donate a unit of blood at each appointment. You will need to drink extra liquid, load up on iron-rich foods, and even take an iron supplement to make sure that you are not anemic and will not develop anemia before surgery.

Transfusion using your own blood guarantees that there will be no errors in cross-matching and that the donor is free of disease.

What happens if you don't need a transfusion? Then the hospital will use your blood for other purposes.

What's crucial: You have eliminated a major potential risk.

430 Keep munchies on your bedside table to lure doctors and nurses.

If you want to guarantee that doctors and nurses visit you frequently, keep cookies or candy on your bedside table. It's a lot more convenient for hospital staff than the cafeteria or the nearest vending machine, and their frequent visits will give you or members of your family the opportunity to ask questions and get answers, or just get more water, pain pills, or have your pillows fluffed.

431 Wear goggles when working with tools.

If you are working in your house or garden, wear protective goggles. Rust specks or other debris that get into your eyes can send you to the emergency room in extreme pain and with possible cornea damage. Regular eyeglasses aren't safe enough because they don't offer protection on the sides.

432 Avoid splinters—especially dangerous for diabetics!

Splinters can get infected easily. Splinters in your feet are especially dangerous because feet contain lots of sweat glands that create an ideal warm, moist environment for bacteria to multiply.

To avoid nasty splinters, wear shoes when you are in your yard or on a wooden deck. Wear gloves when you are working with wood or metal, or are in your garden.

433 Stay away from hospitals and emergency rooms in July.

That's when interns start working. These newbies may have graduated medical school and earned the right to put "M.D." after their names, but internship is their first real experience with patients.

If you can, wait until October, when the new interns have had several months of seasoning—on other patients.

434 Pack now for emergencies…

If you think you might ever need an emergency room, pack now. A small "go" bag with your insurance information, a book or magazine, a list of all medications and vitamins or supplements you take, glucose meter, test strips, lancets, an acceptable snack and a bottle of water, $50 in small bills, important friends' or relatives' phone numbers, a disposable cell phone, an extra house key, a very warm sweater and socks (hospitals and test rooms are kept notoriously freezing to prevent the spread of bacteria), and a change of underwear are all wise inclusions. Just like an expectant mother's "It's time, honey" bag, yours should be immediately grabbable and should contain all the necessary and desirable things you'll wish you had with you—either as you're hurried into an ambulance, or as you sit and fidget in the ER.

435 …And a larger bag for a longer stay.

In addition to the things in your small "go" bag, I recommend some items to make your hospital stay more comfortable: A small framed photograph of your family or pet, moisturizer and lip gloss or makeup, a hairbrush and comb, dental floss, toothbrush, toothpaste, a nightgown or pajamas, T-shirt, perhaps even a Bible or religious book. (Sometimes hospitals provide these amenities, sometimes they don't. And you'll be sure to have the brands you like.)

I also recommend a playground whistle, the "nuclear attention option" discussed in Tip 443. It's crucial if you've been admitted alone.

436 Know what to leave at home.

Unfortunately, theft happens. A friend's wallet and credit cards were stolen while she was waiting for the EMS ambulance. Another friend's wallet went missing somewhere in an emergency room.

To avoid these disasters, leave all valuable jewelry at home and hide it before the EMS arrives. And do the same with your money and credit cards. Of course, hiding all your precious possessions depends on how much you are in control, and whether you have a friend or family member nearby. If you have 10 minutes, you can always hide things in a shopping bag in the nearest closet. Write youself a note or send yourself an email to remind you of what's hidden where.

437 Know how to reach hospital staff.

Before the staff leaves your bedside, know the location of the nurse's bell and whether you can reach it easily.

It's also useful to know the name of the hospital's patient-services coordinator (or similar title) and how to reach him/her.

438 Save the antibacterial soap for special occasions.

All the antibacterial detergents and soaps being sold today have their effects on bacteria: The few survivors are breeding more resistant strains. It's not necessary—in fact, it's not desirable—to use anything stronger than regular soaps or detergents. Save the antibacterial stuff for when you have a cut or other open wound that really requires disinfecting. The product will be much more effective because the bacteria haven't been able to "practice" against it.

439 Be a hospital snob...and research your choices carefully.

Whenever you have the choice, opt for a hospital that must compete for consumer health care dollars. The best ER doctors in Mooseknuckle or even Cincinnati will not have seen as many patients with your problem as their counterparts in Chicago or Los Angeles. At a small-town hospital that's the only game in town, you have the advantage of being known to the staff; but your own physician would also know you at a larger facility that probably has more experience and resources to benefit you. It's not snobbery to choose the hospital that has the best reputation...it's smart strategizing.

440 How come the emergency room is taking so darn long?

As you sit and wait in the emergency room, keep repeating to yourself, "This is a good sign." After initial assessment, patient care is prioritized based on the nature of the illness or injury. Life-threatening, critical-care situations are always given top priority—and usually that order is shifting constantly as unexpected patients arrive.

So if breathing or bleeding emergencies are ahead of you in line, it's a sort of blessing in disguise: You are in better shape than those folks. However, you have the right to ask about an estimated time for treatment.

441 Don't flip out if the emergency room is full.

Don't panic if you arrive at the emergency room and find almost every chair filled. Not all of those people are actually ahead of you. Factors you never considered may affect how long it takes to receive treatment. A patient might need a specific room whose equipment is already in use. Procedures like X rays, lab tests, and scans take time to be processed, and patients and their families have to wait. Specialists may have to be consulted and have to examine a patient. And some people could be waiting for admission to the hospital. So just find yourself a chair—and don't panic until you have all the facts.

442 Beauty and delightfulness are good ER strategies.

It's not fair, but it's true. Humans respond better and more quickly to more attractive people. Since it's too late to pick better-looking ancestors, raise your attractiveness factor by being as delightful as possible to the ER staff. That doesn't mean being a doormat or sucking up, but it does mean being as polite and pleasant as you can manage—even when you're sick and scared. Be sure that anyone accompanying you is also polite, but direct. Of course the people most urgently in need of care will be seen first, but wouldn't it be great to go to the head of the line of everyone at your level of need? Be someone the staff won't cringe at, and your calls for a nurse may be (appropriately) prioritized.

443 The one-and-only nuclear attention option.

Your real, sincere-but-not-considered-emergency calls for assistance or attention may be ignored by overworked staffers, or you may be left in a room with no one checking back on you after someone has downshifted your crisis. If you've been foresighted enough to put a whistle (even a cheap plastic coach's whistle will do) into your grab-and-go bag (see Tip 435), you will have a way to reach past the curtains and down the halls to alert a staffer.

Warning: This is for true emergencies only, to be used if you have been admitted alone and have no one else to send or speak for you. You can do this only once—any more and you'll be considered obnoxious.

You'll also scare the heck out of the cardiac patient on the adjacent gurney, and you should expect your whistle to be confiscated after you've tooted it. But because nurse-call buttons sometimes don't work, and some ER staffers have been at their jobs so long that they forget there's a patient with feelings attached to your paperwork, having a last-resort strategy to summon attention from a distance is as easy as forethought.

444 Your Health-Care Proxy I: Every person with diabetes needs one.

A health-care proxy is a legal document that you absolutely, positively must have just in case you are unable—even temporarily—to make treatment decisions for yourself. Laws vary from state to state. In some states, only your health-care agent—not a family member—has the authority to make these crucial decisions.

445 Your Health-Care Proxy II: Decisions, decisions...

As long as you are a competent adult over the age of 18, you can appoint a health-care agent (who also must be competent and over the age of 18) by signing a health-care proxy. You don't need a lawyer or a notary, just two adult witnesses, neither of whom can be your agent or alternate agent.

446 Your Health-Care Proxy III: Make your wishes clear.

You can and should indicate your specific orders on the proxy form, including your choice of life support if you are in a coma, treatment if you have a terminal illness, and whether you want artificial nutrition or hydration, and under what conditions.

If your agent does not know your wishes, he/she is legally required to act in your own best interest. However, you are much wiser to discuss your wishes in advance.

447 Your Health-Care Proxy IV: Want to change it?

Your proxy isn't written in stone. If you want to cancel it, change your health-care agent, or change your instructions, just fill out a new form.

You can also direct that this proxy expires on a specific date, or if certain events take place. Otherwise, your proxy will be valid indefinitely.

If you choose your spouse as your health-care agent or alternate and you become divorced or legally separated, the appointment is canceled automatically. If you want your former spouse to remain your agent, state this on your current form and date it or complete a new form naming him or her.

448 Your Health-Care Proxy V: Make six copies.

You need at least six copies of your health-care proxy. *Deliver them to…*

1. Your health-care agent

2. Your doctor (or doctors)

3. Your attorney

4. At least one family member or close friend

And also…

5. Keep one with all your other important papers—but not in your safe-deposit box because no one else may be able to get it.

6. Keep one in your wallet next to your driver's license or insurance card, in case you have an accident and are admitted to the hospital, or even have outpatient surgery.

449 Always get a second opinion for a serious condition.

Fewer than one in four Americans gets a second opinion from another specialist, which is a shame because these visits are often covered by insurance. Second opinions can protect you if the first specialist made a diagnostic error or test results are not conclusive. If the specialist uses words like "We're not sure" or "You seem…," get a second opinion.

Best bet: Consult a physician in a related field, like a gastroenterologist or an oncologist who does not perform surgery. Make it clear that you are seeing this specialist for a second opinion only. (You can always change your mind and use him/her for longer-term care.)

450 Sometimes third opinions are necessary.

If the first two opinions disagree, you may need a third. (In that case, many insurance companies and Medicare and Medicaid cover the third opinion.)

Get a clear consensus that the suggested treatment is the best one for you. Most conditions can wait a few weeks while you weigh all the options.

451 Trust your instincts.

You are the world's greatest expert on your body, personality, and lifestyle. A treatment that is right for someone else may be wrong for you. Let your doctor's opinion guide your decision, but not overrule it.

452 Discuss alternative therapies with your primary-care provider.

Many medical groups are expanding into alternative medicine and, in larger cities and their suburbs, your primary physician may be your best guide. Chiropractic, acupuncture, and physical therapy are usually covered by your insurance provider and may help you.

453 Vital signs may not be vital in your case.

Ask your doctor whether your vital signs really need to be checked every four hours. (If not, you may be able to get a good night's rest, even in the hospital.)

454 Personalize your hospital space.

Brighten your little corner with flowers, photos of family and pets, and your kids' artwork. Not only will they cheer you up, they'll also send a message to the hospital staff that you are a real person, not just a chart.

455 Create your very own DO NOT DISTURB sign.

This advice comes directly from my primary care provider…

Bring a Magic Marker, adhesive tape, and some paper with you. With your doctor's permission, make a DO NOT DISTURB sign and tape it on your door. It can be removed as needed, but this way you've got a chance to get some rest!

456 Have a steady stream of visitors.

Visitors influence how the hospital staff treats you. If you don't have visitors, your health providers may be inclined to pay less attention to you. Visitors will advocate for you and send the message that other people care about you.

457 Know your numbers...

Before you leave for the hospital, jot down these numbers and keep them handy...

> •**Your blood pressure**—yes, they check it often, but it helps if you know your normal range

> •**Your hemoglobin A1C and microalbumin**—especially if you have (or are at risk for) kidney disease

> *Asthmatics:* Know your peak flow. (You should be testing at home.) It lets the hospital choose the best treatment for you.

458 ...And your other test results.

If you have it, bring a copy of your most recent EKG, especially if you are at risk for cardiovascular disease. Your family doctor should have some scaled-down extra copies in your file. You may not know how to read your EKG—many patients don't—but the hospital staff will, and they will have something to compare with any new tests.

459 Don't forget this one more thing to bring.

If you have glaucoma, bring your eye drops with you. Approximately two dozen different glaucoma eye drop medications are prescribed in the U.S., and my primary-care provider says that hospitals often don't have all of them. However, some hospitals still won't let you bring any drugs from home. If there's time, check first to see if that's the case, and ask your doctor so that you can bring your own glaucoma eye drops.

460 Learn everyone's name.

When you address doctors and nurses by name, they know you know who they are and legally, it makes them responsible for any problems on their watch. Also, treating the staff like individuals, rather than their job descriptions, gets you better care.

461 Before you start treatment, do this...

Ask your doctor about side effects, benefits and risks, and recommended reading, including reliable websites.

Bring a relative or friend with you for support and ask him/her to take notes for you, or bring a tape recorder so that you can replay the doctor's diagnosis and instructions as often as necessary.

462 Get explanations.

Make your questions more palatable by saying, "I don't understand. Would you please explain that more simply?" If you don't understand the medical terminology, as many patients don't, ask your doctor to explain every word.

463 Know what you're being given—and why.

Hospital "accidents" happen. Minimize the risk that they happen to you. Know the pills and other treatments that the nurses and technicians give you. *Ask them these questions…*

> Who are you? (name and job title)
> What is this?
> Who ordered this?
> Why?
> What is it supposed to do?
> Are you trained to administer this? (Sometimes nurses and technicians cover

for each other.)

464 Make sure they wash their hands before they touch you.

According to recent statistics, tens of thousands of Americans die each year from infections they acquired as hospital patients. The worst infections—post-surgical sepsis in the bloodstream—resulted in much longer hospital stays and increased risk of death.

One simple request can minimize your risk. Say to any staffer who comes near you, "I'm terrified of hospital infections."

If they don't take the hint, be blunt: "Please wash your hands before you touch me."

465 Avoid hospital-acquired infections.

According to the Centers for Disease Control and Prevention's annual *National and State Healthcare-Associated Infections Progress Report* (2014 data reported in 2016), there were 722,000 hospital-acquired infections (HAIs) in U.S. acute-care hospitals. About 75,000 patients (over 10%!) with these HAIs died during their hospitalizations.

A cover story in the February 2014 magazine *Managed Care*, quoting a recent study in *Journal of the American Medical Association Internal Medicine* found that nearly 441,000 patients contract one of five HAIs each year, about half of which are avoidable. The five most common, costly, and preventable hospital infections are surgical site infections (SSI), central-line associated bloodstream infections (CLABSI), catheter-associated urinary tract infections (CAUTI), ventilator-associated pneumonia (VAP), and Clostridium difficile (C. diff) infections (CDI). Methicillin-resistant Staphylococcus aureus (MRSA) is a subcategory of SSIs and CLABSIs.

Leah Binder, president and CEO of Leapfrog Group, an organization that issues semiannual hospital-safety scores, stated graphically that U.S. hospitals are infecting a population the size of Atlanta every year.

To protect yourself, find out the hospital's infection rate; it should be below 6%. If your doctor doesn't know, talk to the hospital's infection-control officer—every hospital must have one. If the infection rate is higher, ask your doctor to admit you to another hospital.

466 Keep your dignity in the hospital.

No one said you had to wear a hospital-issue johnny, one of those unpleasant short gowns that are open all the way up the back. They are uncomfortable, embarrassing, and dehumanizing. Bring your own PJs, robe, underwear, and slippers. Men, your favorite T-shirt and briefs or boxers are fine. And women, your favorite sexy nightgown can cheer you up. Express your individuality— your self-esteem really needs it now!

467 Check your surgeon's and anesthesiologist's track records.

Make sure that your surgeon and anesthesiologist don't have an ugly record of malpractice suits. States vary in making this information available to ordinary people, but doctors or lawyers can access it easily. Your best bet is to ask your family doctor or another doctor you trust about these specialists' track records.

468 Have a presurgery discussion with your anesthesiologist.

Several days before your surgery, ask your anesthesiologist these questions…
What drug will you use?
Is it all right to use with the drugs I am taking? Go through your list.
How is it administered?
Why did you select it?
Is it recommended for people with diabetes?
What are the risks? What are the side effects?
It may sound paranoid, but it's a smart way to protect yourself.

469 Try for an early release…

Sounds like prison, doesn't it? But home healing is usually better and faster. Many medical treatments can be continued at your home, and there's much less risk of hospital-acquired infection.

470 ...But fight premature discharge.

If you can't keep food or liquid down, can't go to the bathroom without help, have pain that can't be controlled by pills, or feel disoriented or unsteady, you are not ready to go home.

If the hospital still tries to discharge you, insist on talking to your doctor. If your doctor can't get your stay extended, talk to the hospital's discharge planner or patient advocate.

Go up the ladder. Your next step is contacting your insurance carrier and the hospital administrator. If you are on Medicaid or Medicare, hospitals must give you a toll-free number to call to appeal their decisions.

471 Get clear, concise discharge instructions.

Whether it's from the emergency room or from the hospital, get clear discharge instructions. *They should include...*

- Special eating and drinking instructions.
- Bathing or showering instructions.
- Necessary prescriptions.
- Any changes in the drugs you are taking, and why.
- Follow-up doctors' appointments that you need to make.
- Any limitations on physical activity, including on work.
- Any dangerous "red flags" that make it necessary to call 911 and return to the ER.

472 Don't forget your escort service.

Your discharge instructions probably include an escort (provided by you), without whom you may not be permitted to leave the ER or hospital.

In many states, your escort must be at least 21 and provide ID.

When you arrive home, ask your escort to stay for at least an hour or two—just in case. Your escort's staying with you—and checking up on you—may prevent your being readmitted.

473 "Please autograph my leg."

Surgeons operating on the wrong side of the body are grist for the tabloids. These blunders are rare, but they happen often enough that the American Academy of Orthopaedic Surgeons has advised its members to initial the surgery site beforehand. Ask your surgeon to mark the site and initial it—in case of trouble, this has more legal standing than your marking the area with lipstick or a pen.

474 Be the second or third surgery in the morning.

During the first surgery of the day, the surgeon and the surgical team are often still warming up, not quite up to peak performance. The second or third slot is much better, and you'll still get your immediate postoperative care during the day shift, when the nursing staff is at full strength.

475 Get walking ASAP.

Walking as soon as possible reduces the risk of developing dangerous blood clots in your legs or pneumonia from inactivity. If you need support, ask a nurse, friend, or relative to lend an arm. And ask for special elastic stockings to improve your circulation while you are recovering if you are overweight or have varicose veins.

476 Prevent deep-vein thrombosis (DVT).

Deep-vein thrombosis (DVT) refers to blood clots that develop in the legs, often as a result of immobility in bed. But up to eight weeks after hospitalization or surgery they can travel up to the lungs (pulmonary emboli) and become potentially fatal.

Ask your doctor what is being done to prevent DVT; compression stockings and blood thinners are often prescribed.

Warning signs: Leg pain or redness, problems breathing. Call your doctor immediately!

477 Know who's in charge.

Several specialists may examine you while you're in the hospital. Make sure that one doctor coordinates your treatment so that the chance of overlapping or conflicting orders is minimized. Ideally, your primary care physician or a colleague should visit you every day.

478 Avoid hospital overcharges I: Know what's covered.

If it's not an emergency, check your insurance policy to find out exactly what it will cover and how much it will pay. Read the "Exceptions and Exclusions" section over and over because it spells out what your policy will not cover.

After your body, your bottom line is at greatest risk in a hospital. Imagine being billed $129 for a "mucus recovery system." Believe it or not, that's hospital-speak for a box of tissues! One middle-aged man who had hip surgery was charged for a crib and newborn blood tests!

Steve Brill's February 20, 2013, *Time* magazine 11-page cover story, "Bitter Pill," describes obscene markups on many hospital charges, such as $1.50

for a generic acetaminophen (headache) tablet, when you can buy an entire 100-tablet bottle for $2 to $3, $18 for one Accu-Check blood-glucose test strip that you can buy for around 55 cents, or $283 for a simple chest X-ray for which the hospital routinely gets less than $25 when it treats a Medicare patient.

And in 2014, National Nurses United, the largest U.S. nurses' union, released data from its 2011 study, finding that the 100 most expensive hospitals charged 765% over their costs, or $765 for every $100. In 2014, hospital daily charges ranged from $1,294 (South Dakota) to $3,344 (Oregon), nearly three times higher.

Estimates on hospital overcharges run well over $10 billion a year, with an average of $1,500 per hospital stay. Many experts believe that many of these charges are deliberate. *Here are more tips to help you avoid getting clipped and having your credit destroyed…*

479 Avoid hospital overcharges II: All about room charges.

Call the hospital's billing department and find out exactly what the room charges cover. Better yet, ask them to fax you a list. You may need this ammunition. If they're charging you for soap and a toothbrush, bring your own!

480 Avoid hospital overcharges III: Your doctor can help.

Ask your doctor about how much your treatment will cost and whether you can bring and use your own prescription drugs to avoid paying for the hospital's medications.

481 Avoid hospital overcharges IV: Are the doctors in-network?

Make sure that all the doctors who will be treating you—the anesthesiologist, the surgeon, the pathologist, the rehabilitation specialist—participate in your insurance plan. If not, your charges may be astronomical!

482 Avoid hospital overcharges V: Keep track.

Keep a record of medications, tests, and treatments or ask a relative or friend to do it for you. You'll want to check these charges against the bills when they arrive.

483 Avoid hospital overcharges VI: Don't pay the bill yet.

Regardless of what the staff tells you, never pay the bill before you leave the hospital.

484 Avoid hospital overcharges VII: Get an itemized bill.

Compare the bill to your record of treatment. Read it very carefully. If anything looks vague, demand an itemized bill—every state requires hospitals to do so.

Ask for your medical records, too, and compare them with your bill to check whether or not you received the medications and treatments you have been billed for.

485 Avoid hospital overcharges VIII: Go to the top.

Hospital billing departments hope that you will cave in and pay unquestionably. Don't. Write to the hospital administrator, then the hospital president and—if necessary—every single individual on the board of trustees. (You can find their names on the hospital's website.) These people all know that bad publicity can cost them big bucks in contributions.

486 Call in the cavalry!

You have some powerful watchdog organizations on your side. If the hospital stonewalls you or threatens to ruin your credit rating, try these, and be firm…

- **American Hospital Association** (your state's chapter or the national organization) (AHA.org)
- **National Health Care Anti-Fraud Association** (NHCAA.org)
- **Blue Cross/Blue Shield Division of Special Investigations** (Bluecross. com, organized by state)
- **Your insurance provider**

CHAPTER 5

Exercise

487   Any exercise you do is good.

OK, this is a baby step from your sedentary lifestyle to something more active. And you may need many more baby steps to really get moving.

Bottom line: Any exercise you do will help you. You'll start seeing the results in as little as one month.

488   Just don't call it exercise.

Many of us have a hatred of exercise that dates back to grade school, when we were the chubby, slow, ungraceful kids who were always chosen last for sports teams.

Nevertheless, physical activity is a crucial component of good diabetes care. There's a simple solution. Find something you like to do. Stroll through city streets and parks. Wander through museums or malls with a friend. Go for a bike ride or play volleyball with your kids or grandkids. Go out dancing or put on some music and dance at home.

You can even walk around your house—set a kitchen timer.

The winning strategy? Feeling "Hey, this isn't so bad; I can stick with this." Or maybe even, "I feel good; I'll do a little more of this tomorrow."

Just don't call it exercise!

489   Start slowly to stay successful.

Start very slowly. If you're out of shape, start with a five- or 10-minute walk. Work at your own pace and establish a daily commitment that's best for you. The important thing is that you start and keep going.

490 Be a creative dog walker.

Get an extra workout when you walk your dog. Keep the leash short and step away from it until you can feel the pull. Bend over slowly until your head is in line with your waist, forming a right angle with your legs. Then straighten up slowly. Repeat four or five times, then move on and bend again. This bending and straightening stretches your latissimus dorsi, the muscles in your back between your ribs and your hips.

491 Walk around in circles.

This tip works well for city dwellers.

Do you enjoy walking, but hate being stopped by traffic lights? You won't lose momentum if you go around the block. In most cities, three circuits measure a little over one mile.

Increase your workout by finding a block with one uphill and one downhill side.

492 Reward yourself!

Motivate yourself to walk or bike instead of taking public transport by banking your carfare. Put the money in a clear glass jar or bowl so that seeing it will inspire you to add to the kitty.

When the container is full—or every month or so—reward yourself with a little nonfood treat, such as a massage, a movie, a bunch of fresh flowers or a piece of clothing that says you're trimming down! Then start the cycle again. Massages are a stress-reducing indulgence enjoyed by both men and women.

493 Reorganize your kitchen.

Make your kitchen less convenient to get more of a workout you don't have to think about.

Put items you use every day—like coffee filters, sugar substitutes, your most-used pots and pans—on the highest and lowest shelves. If you need to bend, stretch or climb on a step stool several times a day, you're exercising without realizing it.

494 Keep it easy…keep it fun!

You probably know that regular exercise reduces your risk of cardiovascular disease by 30%. But did you know that your workout doesn't have to be hard? Brisk walking for 30 minutes at least five days a week will give you the same reduction in risk as more vigorous exercise such as running, with less wear and tear on your hips, knees, and ankles.

495 Use a bed or a chair.

Is it difficult for you to move around? You can do many exercises lying down or sitting in a chair. As your body becomes more flexible and you develop more strength and energy, increase the number of repetitions you do and the length of your workout sessions.

496 Let the water help you exercise.

Many overweight people excel at swimming because their bodies are naturally buoyant and they don't have to fight gravity. Their knees, hips, and ankles don't hurt as much, either.

If swimming laps bores you, try a water aerobics class, or do water exercises on your own.

497 Take advantage of tax-deductions.

You can deduct the cost of your gym membership and of any exercise classes as a medical expense on your federal and local income-tax returns. Note, however, that the total amount of your medical expenses must exceed 10% of adjusted gross income to qualify as a deduction.

Get a letter from your doctor stating that the gym membership and classes are necessary for weight loss and diabetes care, and attach copies of the letter to your tax returns.

You will have to list this amount on your Form 1040 Schedule A line 1 as part of your medical and dental expenses, enter your adjusted gross income on line 2, multiply this amount by 10%—but if either you or your spouse is 65 or older, multiply this amount by 7½%. Enter this amount on line 3, subtract it from line 1, and enter this number on line 4. Unfortunately, if line 3 is more than line 1, you must enter 0.

498 Try before you buy.

Human nature being what it is, we all start off with the best of intentions. We'll buy exercise equipment—also tax-deductible as a medical expense with a doctor's letter—and use it faithfully, or join a gym and go faithfully.

But then reality or inertia intrudes, and that exercise equipment becomes an expensive clothes rack and the gym membership becomes just another card in your wallet.

Save your money! Try a one-month membership at the gym, or a one-month rental of that jazzy exercise machine. See how often you use them before you buy them.

499 **Fidget!**

Make use of spare minutes and rev up your metabolism without thinking about it. *All of these count as exercise…*

Waiting for the elevator? Do heel or toe raises or contract your glutes.

Watching the clock in a waiting room? Sit up straight in your chair, raise your legs, and do leg extensions.

Waiting to cross the street? March or jog in place.

500 **Stop using the remote control.**

Move around the room. At least, get up to change the TV program or adjust the volume. Movement is cumulative. Don't be a couch potato!

501 **Ask your doctor.**

You've probably heard that you should consult a physician before undertaking any exercise program. *However,* make sure that you ask your doctor what he/ she knows about the particular form of exercise you would like to partake in, and if it could be harmful to you in any way.

502 **Try weight training.**

Weight training builds lean muscle mass. That speeds up your metabolic rate, which helps burn fat and carbohydrates.

Some forms of weight training can be hard on your joints. The least-taxing system is Super Slow, which requires fewer repetitions to achieve the same results, while not putting so much stress on your joints.

503 **Explore yoga, tai chi and qi gong…**

Yoga, tai chi, and qi gong emphasize flexibility and build stamina and endurance. The slower pace is beneficial for older, sedentary people with diabetes. All three systems are designed to open up the flow of chi (life energy) and to improve breathing, which oxygenates the blood, increasing circulation and your metabolic rate.

504 **…But beware the martial arts class.**

Many martial arts programs aren't very aerobic. If your class emphasizes learning techniques, you can spend a lot of time waiting your turn to perform the action. "Martial arts" is about combat and, like combat, can often mean long periods of waiting, followed by short bursts of intense activity, stressing different body parts. Punching and kicking place more stress on your knees, hips, wrists, and shoulders. Throwing and grappling will stress your hips. The part of your body receiving the most workout will vary from style to style.

If you think the challenge of kung-fu fighting will keep you committed to getting fit, be sure to investigate before you join a class.

505 Remember that black belt can mean red flag!

Avoid any martial arts school that *guarantees* you a black belt or wants you to commit to a long-term contract. Ask to watch a class or two to get some idea of the activity and of the teacher's ability. If you are refused, go elsewhere. If you are told that the techniques are "too dangerous for the casual or uncommitted observer"...run—do not walk—to the nearest exit!

506 Try out a few videos.

OK, you don't have the time or money to go to a gym. Or your body embarrasses you.

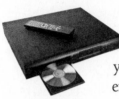

If you have a DVD player, you have hundreds of options. There are many exercise programs to try out in the privacy of your home. Borrow DVDs from a friend or from the library before you buy them. Get to know a certain teacher or activity you enjoy (Zumba, Jazzercise, yoga, etc.), then purchase one or two discs online...and have them delivered straight to your home.

Photo: GeorgePeters

507 Indulge in your dreams of ballet dancing.

Ballet class isn't just for kids...the disciplined classes work well for adults too. Beginners' ballet emphasizes balance and coordination and develops flexibility, grace, and posture. Take a class at your local Y, or check out a DVD.

508 Try belly dancing.

Here is an exercise where generous curves are a distinct advantage. You can be overweight and still feel very sensual, which should motivate you to continue this sexy, satisfying exercise.

509 Vary your exercise routine.

Boredom is the enemy of self-discipline. We get tired of the workout routine, and soon we just quit.

Fight the inevitable monotony by varying your exercise routine. Racewalk one day, climb stairs another, go swimming or dancing later in the week. Variety will keep your interest sparked.

510 Pilates without the machines.

The Pilates system offers its disciples long, lean, beautifully toned muscles—strong, but not bulging. But Pilates machines cost hundreds of dollars and occupy lots of space.

Some excellent Pilates programs now available on video are designed to be used without the machines. Instead, you perform the low-impact exercises on a mat very, very slowly, so that you get the gain without the pain.

511 Have a bad-weather alternative.

Don' let rain or snow dampen your plans. Find an indoor exercise alternative for nasty weather. Some of the best for combining pleasure with exercise are mall walking and visiting museums.

512 Get a pedometer…

This lightweight little gadget can inspire you just by clocking how much walking you do every day. Every step counts, whether it's housework, doing errands, or racewalking.

If you need encouragement, keep track of your weekly distances and try to increase them every week or every other week. Or calculate the distance from your home to some marvelous destination—New York? San Francisco? London? Paris? Samarkand? The length of Hadrian's Wall?—and log how long it'll take you to get there. Keep a map and a Magic Marker stuck to the fridge!

Before you buy your pedometer, make sure that it will not stop counting if you stop moving for more than 15 minutes, and make sure that you can return or exchange it within two weeks if you find it uncomfortable or inaccurate. Just remember that pedometers give you an *approximate* measurement, based on body movement (most pedometers attach to your waist). Most claim a 5% error, but the distance counted could be as high as 10% off.

You can also download a pedometer app to your smartphone. Again, it's not perfect, but whenever you have your phone, it'll record how far you go.

513 …But stop and think before you buy a fitness monitor.

These are a bit more involved than your simple pedometer—counting calories, recording heart rate (which determines the intensity of your exercise), monitoring sleep patterns, plus more. They can set goals, along with tracking steps and distances. They come in many models (with funky names such as Fitbit, Jawbone, Moov, Misfit and Pebble) and prices, ranging from $50 to close to $500. But before you pull out your wallet, ask yourself how committed you would be to using a fitness monitor. Will simply having it and wearing it motivate you to exercise more, or will it just wind up on your night table (which, researchers found, happens to one-third users)?

Be aware, too, that according to a recent study out of the Cleveland Clinic, many wrist-worn fitness monitors were found to be inaccurate and misreported the wearer's heart rate, sometimes with serious consequences. You might be better off checking your pulse periodically using your watch's second hand.

514 Procrastinating doesn't pay off.

"Tomorrow and tomorrow" isn't just the beginning of a *Macbeth* soliloquy; it sums up many people's attitude toward exercise. Starting your exercise plan "tomorrow" is great, but when the sun rises, tomorrow becomes today, and somehow your plan never gets off the drawing board.

515 Enjoy the delights of dancing.

Dancing is a feel-good, total-body exercise. Many forms are good for a lifetime—ballroom or freestyle, swing, folk dancing, English or Scottish country dancing, salsa, and line or square dancing. The best part is that the level of participation is up to you. Some forms are strenuous; the country dance "Strip the Willow" is best reserved for Iron Man competitors.

Many kinds of dance do not require partners, a blessing for single people, and many types of dance have clubs and weekly events in many U.S. cities.

Note: If you need or want to take lessons, be sure to read the fine print (especially at the big dance school chains). Don't be conned into expensive yearlong—or even "lifetime"—contracts. Many companies offer three-month lesson programs, which should be enough to master the movements you need for steady practice.

516 Be an Easy Rider.

Back problems? Painful knees or hips? You can still get the exercise benefits of bicycle riding with a recumbent bike. This exercise machine lets you lie comfortably on your back and pedal away. You get a minimal-impact workout that improves your circulation and burns calories without stressing your joints.

517 Grab a broomstick.

You can use a household broom or mop as an exercise tool. Wrap your fingers around the ends of the stick and turn to the right as far as you can comfortably. Then turn to the left as far as you can. The stick provides a little weight and momentum, so you'll get more of a workout. This exercise is a wonderful waist-whittler. Do this for 16 repetitions per side and work your way up.

518 Clean your house.

Think of all the bending, stretching, and reaching you do when you dust, sweep, vacuum, and scrub. You may not think of this as exercise, but it is. An hour of heavy housecleaning will burn as many calories as an hour of race-walking. (You may want to check your blood glucose afterward.)

519 Tend your garden.

You dig, plant, water, prune, harvest. It's a very pleasant aerobic workout. And being out in the sun provides vitamin D, necessary for building and protecting your bones. (But please wear a protective hat and sunblock for extended periods.)

520 Pace!

Your cordless or cell phone can help you exercise. Don't just sit there when you're talking—pace up and down, back and forth. You'll get some exercise without realizing it.

521 Lengthen your stride.

To increase benefits from exercising, lengthen your stride when you walk. Just lengthening it by five or six inches will do the trick. Your posture will improve, too.

522 Perk up your workout.

If you can't go without your morning cup of joe, exercising soon after could give your workout a boost.

In a recent study out of the University of Georgia, people who consumed about a coffee cup's worth of caffeine before their workouts experienced less exercise-caused muscle pain during their exertions. Researchers speculate that the caffeine could boost exercise endurance.

523 Bed exercise I: Leg raises.

Lying in bed, raise one leg slowly as high as you can, toes pointed, to a count of 10. Hold for a count of 10, then lower to a count of 10. Then do the same with the other leg. Keep alternating and do five raises each side. Over time, increase the number of leg raises gradually. Keep on increasing the number of leg raises until it just begins to hurt. That's when the effect is greatest.

524 Bed exercise II: Hip rolls.

Lying on your back, swing one leg across your body as far as possible without lifting your hips off the mattress, to a count of five. Hold for a count of five, then swing your leg back to a count of five. Repeat this sequence five times, then switch legs. Work up to five sets of 10 leg swings on each side. (This is a wonderful waist-whittler.)

525 Bed exercise III: Back stretch plus.

Lying on your back, pull your knees up to your chest. Hold for a count of five. Straighten out your legs and lower them to a count of 10. Using this slow count, repeat this exercise until you cannot complete one.

As you get more flexible, make this exercise harder by extending your legs over your head and rolling up onto your shoulders, then swinging your legs downward in a long arc to a count of 10. When you can do the whole exercise as a unit, you will stretch your back, tighten your abs, and strengthen your lower back all in one exercise. Gradually increase the number of repetitions, and also lengthen the count for each part of the exercise.

526 Bed exercise IV: Build bridges.

Lying on your back with your arms down at your sides, bend your legs at the knees and push up your buttocks in line with your knees. Hold for a count of 20, tighten your abdominal muscles, then relax. Repeat 10 times, then 20.

527 Bed exercise V: Twinkle toes.

Lying on your back with your arms down at your sides and your legs extended, point your toes ballet-style, then flex your feet, toes pointing up at the ceiling. Point, flex. Point, flex. Keep on repeating. This exercise is designed to stimulate the circulation in your feet and guard against diabetic neuropathy.

528 Bed exercise VI: Run in place.

Lying in bed, with your knees bent and your feet flat on the bed, run in place. See how long you can keep this up. Increase your "running" time every day!

529 Office exercise: First, check your desk.

For all exercises at your desk, be sure that your desk is either heavy enough or anchored well enough that you won't move it or tip it over. Be sure that your chair is stable, too.

530 Office exercise I: Push-pull.

This exercise requires a chair with wheels. At your desk, raise your feet slightly off the floor. Use your arms to pull yourself forward, then push backward as far as you can go. If you have room, lean forward as far as possible on the "push" and try to come to a full upright position on the "pull."

531 Office exercise II: Leg raises.

At your desk, raise your legs until they are completely extended straight out in front of you, then lower them. Use the same count as for the leg raises in bed (Tip #523). With your hands at your sides, grip the seat of your chair so that you can't use them to help raise your legs.

532 Office exercise III: Gluteus crunches.

At your desk, extend your legs slightly off the floor. Raise them by clenching your buttocks. Use a count of five to raise, five to hold, and five to lower. Start with a set of five and increase gradually.

533 Office exercise IV: Shoulder rolls.

This exercise is less strenuous than the next one, so always do it first to warm up. Roll your shoulders backward slowly eight times, then forward slowly eight times. Do four or five sets.

This exercise will relieve back and neck strain that frequently accompanies heavy keyboard use, whether computer or musical.

534 Office exercise V: Shoulder circles.

With your arms fully extended, make small circles in the air so that your fingertips are moving only a few inches. Circle forward for a count of 10, hold for a count of 10, and then circle backward for a count of 10. Start with a set of five and increase gradually.

535 Make isometrics work for you.

Isometrics is the exercise technique that pits one set of your body muscles against their opposites. For example, put the heels of your hands together in front of your chest. Try to push one hand toward its opposite side, then reverse. You can also do this exercise with your hands placed over your head. Any way you can work your body's muscles against themselves will increase their strength and, if done long enough and with increasing effort, will help build muscle and increase your metabolism.

536 Remember that soreness = success.

Muscle growth is the result of muscle fiber being stretched and torn so that new muscle fiber grows in. Small wonder that your muscles are sore after a really hard workout, or that most exercise experts advise resting for a day between workouts.

If you feel sore, reward yourself with a long soak in a hot tub. Epsom salts and other mineral treatments help!

537 Music, Maestro!

Did you know that orchestra conductors are extraordinarily long-lived? Their secret? The wonderful cardiovascular workout they get by moving their arms for hours nearly every day.

You'll get a great workout by playing conductor to symphonic music or operas for at least 20 minutes at a time.

538 Lighten up.

Light weights work well for beginning exercisers. You can find them right in your pantry. Cans of soup weighing approximately one pound are easy to wrap your fingers around. When you can do 40 or 50 repetitions of two or three different exercises, it's time to move up to heavier weights.

Note: Anyone with retinopathy or high blood pressure should be very careful about lifting weights. Consult your doctor first!

539 Be inefficient.

Carry your packages and bags of groceries from your car one by one, to make as many trips as possible. This is an easy exercise that doesn't require any advance planning or thinking.

540 Add walking to your driving and riding.

Take a more distant parking space and walk a little more. Make this part of your daily routine. If you use public transportation, get off a few stops before your usual one and walk to your destination.

541 Take advantage of TV commercial breaks.

Don't just sit there or make a beeline for snacks. Walk in place (or run!), do push-ups against the nearest wall, or do squats.

You'll find that you're exercising for at least 10 minutes every hour!

542 Climb the stairway to success.

If you work in an office building or live in an apartment building, you can be a stair climber, rather than using one at the health club. Start by walking up or down only one flight each time instead of using the elevator for the whole trip. Increase your stair climbing by one flight up and one flight down every week. Make sure that you climb up *and* down because you use different muscles for each exercise. Soon you'll be zipping up and down the stairs, avoiding the elevator crush, and giving yourself a wonderful cardiovascular workout.

543 Take a walk after dinner.

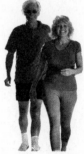

Going for a walk after dinner offers many benefits…
● **It removes you from the kitchen and dining room,** which may tempt you to eat more.
● **It revs up your metabolism when you need it most.**
● **It's a great stress and tension reliever.**
● **It can give you and your partner and/or your kids some uninterrupted time together.**

Photo: FatCamera

544 Grab some light weights.

Stretching is a great way to improve your flexibility and balance and increase your range of motion. Research suggests that stretching with a set of light weights in your hands may bring even better results. Stick to very light weights—one or two pounds—until you become accustomed to the added load.

545 Play a musical instrument.

Yes, this counts as exercise, too. Playing most musical instruments gives you a powerful aerobic payoff. Think of the deep-breathing exercise you get in playing a wind or brass instrument, or the powerful upper-body workout you get in playing the piano, drums, or a string instrument.

546 Play on the floor.

Sit on the floor with your legs spread, back straight. Play jacks or pick-up sticks alone or with your kids. Sit in a chair and pick up marbles of different sizes with your toes. Have fun!

547 Keep your equipment handy.

When you have to plow through your closets to find your exercise gear, you're much less likely to use it consistently. Keep your outfit and equipment in one accessible place so that you'll use them often.

548 You can handle it.

If you can't touch your toes or have other flexibility problems, use the handles on a sturdy chest of drawers or kitchen cabinets to reach lower and lower. These heavy pieces of furniture are very stable and won't move as you reach down farther and farther.

549 Make an investment in your fitness.

Think of fitness as a long-term investment in your life. Just as you put away money in a 401(k) or IRA every year in order to benefit during your retirement, keeping your body moving over the long term will pay off when you are much older.

Why is this important? According to the National Center for Health Statistics, a person who lives to age 65 will live, on average, over 20 more years. Experts say that even slow, low-impact fitness programs can make your biological age 10 years younger than your chronological age.

550 Do the flamingo.

No, it's not a close relative of the Funky Chicken. It's an exercise designed to strengthen your ankles and improve your balance so that you are less likely to take a nasty fall as you get older.

I've named this exercise for its appearance. *Warning*: It's harder than it looks, but the results and protection it will give you are worth the effort.

Stand in a doorway where the floor has no sill and is absolutely flat. Place your palms on either side of the doorway a little lower than shoulder height for balance. Now stand on one leg and raise the other, knee bent. Hold this position for as long as you can; then reverse legs.

At first you may be able to hold the position for only two or three minutes on each side. Work up to five or six if you can.

When this exercise becomes too easy, stop using your hands for balance and keep them at your sides. When that becomes easy, do it on your toes.

551 Spend one hour with a pro.

Just one hour with a personal trainer can be the best investment you make in your exercise routine. In that hour, your trainer should be able to diagnose the areas of your body that need work, teach you the best exercises to achieve the desired results, and the most effective order to do them.

To find a qualified trainer, check these professional groups on the Internet: American College of Sports Medicine (ACSM.org), American Council on Exercise (AceFitness.org), and the National Strength and Conditioning Association (NSCA.com). Then phone the trainers themselves and check at least three of their recent references. And…don't forget…a personal trainer's fees can count as a medical tax deduction.

552 Take this pointed advice.

Standing tall with your knees straight, lift one leg at a time and alternate pointing and flexing your toes for a minute or so. This movement will stretch your hamstrings and help build up your calf muscles (gastrocnemius) and the muscle that lies along the back part of your shin (soleus).

553 Try a treadmill high.

Hitting the treadmill can give you an amphetamine-like lift that lasts for 24 hours. British researchers found that people who ran on a treadmill for 30 minutes produced almost twice as much *phenylethylamine*, a brain chemical similar to amphetamine, than people who were couch potatoes.

554 Create your very own ballet barre.

Improvise an at-home ballet barre for doing forward and backward leg lifts. You won't have to do any work or move any furniture.

Although chairs are often recommended for holding on to, they are too lightweight and slide across the floor, creating a potential hazard. Instead, use the top of your bedroom dresser, which is heavy enough to provide good support.

As a bonus, dressers often have mirrors that you can use to check the posture of your upper body while you do the leg lifts.

555 Combine cardiovascular and resistance exercises.

You'll get more "bang" for your "exercise buck" and save time with exercise that combines cardiovascular workouts with resistance training.

Some of the best: Riding your bike, doing step aerobics, and walking or jogging up and down hills. Is this why most San Franciscans are in such great shape?

556 Stretch at the end, too.

Most people do stretches for warm-ups, before they work out. But stretching at the end of a workout has stronger benefits. Stretching when your muscles are warm actually enhances your flexibility more than stretches at the beginning of your workout, when your muscles are still cold.

557 Stay flexible: Upper body.

Stretching your triceps muscle aids upper-body flexibility. Place a bath towel along your back. Hold the top in your right hand and grasp the bottom in your left hand. Climb up the towel with your left hand as high as you can reach. Alternate hands and repeat.

558 Stay flexible: Lower body.

Stretch the muscles in your lower leg by placing your hands against a wall, elbows straight and arms extended. Bend your right knee and step back one or two feet with your left leg, foot flat on the floor. Hold for a count of eight, working up to 16. Then alternate legs. Do this exercise five times.

559 The 10,000-step prescription.

Exercise gurus urge us to walk at least 10,000 steps every day. This number translates as approximately 4.5 miles (one step = approximately 28.5 inches). *Remember*: Every step counts.

You may want to start by getting some baseline figures. Use a pedometer on two weekdays, plus one weekend day, total the mileage, and divide by three to get your average daily distance in miles. You can then convert this figures to steps, if you like, by multiplying it by 2,200.

If you discover that you are walking only about two miles a day, increase your walking slowly, adding 200 to 300 steps a day.

560 Find your best stride by ignoring it.

Maybe you *don't* need to change your walking or running stride. Your "doing what comes naturally" is safer than consciously changing your stride, which can stress your muscles and joints, thus raising the risk of injury.

561 Lifting weights banishes belly fat.

Belly fat is dangerous. It increases the risk of type 2 diabetes and cardiovascular disease. Over a period of a few months, lifting light weights for multiple repetitions replaces fat with muscle, builds endurance, and reduces the risk of these deadly diseases.

562 Be a silver star.

SilverSneakers classes, offered by many Ys and health clubs, are designed specifically for older exercisers who may have arthritis or other health problems. The aerobic and strength exercises are paced gently but effectively for people over the age of 55.

SilverSneakers programs are available in more than 13,000 participating locations. Group exercise classes are generally provided by your health plan at no additional cost.

SilverSneakers FLEX programs feature more than 50 unique classes, such as...

- **Line dancing and Latin-style dancing**
- **Indoor and outdoor boot camps**
- **Walking groups**

This benefit is covered by several Medicare plans and select private insurers.

563 Slower walking works!

Just getting out there is good for you, and it turns out that it's not the speed, but the distance that burns calories and pounds. Think of the tortoise and the hare, smile, and keep on walking.

564 Where walkers beat runners.

Surprise! Recent research published in the journal *Arteriosclerosis, Thrombosis, and Vascular Biology* reveals that brisk walking delivers similar (in some cases better) risk reductions in hypertension, cholesterol, diabetes and coronary heart disease as running, with less injury and strain.

565 Newbies can profit from interval training.

Short bursts of high-intensity exercise, called "interval training," are proving to be the best exercise for balancing blood glucose. Don't be put off by the term "interval training." It just means alternating between two minutes of moderate walking and 20 seconds of rapid striding. Repeating this exercise for 10 minutes, three times a week, is enough to glean results.

566 Escalator strategy: Walk while you ride.

You can get more of a workout by walking up the escalator than climbing a flight of stairs. That's because the treads on escalators are so much higher. Walking up the escalator burns seven times more calories than standing still, and you'll get to your floor in only half the time.

567 Go mall walking.

Warm, light, and safe in the winter, cool in the summer, and always dry, malls beat running tracks hands down. Whether you join a group or go it alone, mall walking offers a pleasant way to exercise, and you can measure your progress by how far around the mall you can go.

568 Follow some marching orders.

Walking briskly to poetry in your head can really stimulate you and inspire you to do just a little bit more. I like doing this to "Disobedience," a cute poem by Winnie the Pooh author AA. Milne, which begins: James James/Morrison Morrison/Weatherby George Dupree/ Took great care of his mother/Though he was only three…The beat certainly calls for swinging your arms, and you don't have to memorize all six verses, although it's a fun little ditty to know. (An old friend used to fence competitively to this poem.)

569 Do it in the moonlight.

Summer evenings are an ideal time for exercising. The temperature has cooled down, and racewalking and running are much more comfortable.

Take advantage of this special time of lingering twilights to take longer-than-usual walks with your partner, family or friends. Make plans for barbecues, picnics, and parties.

570 Yoga may fight serious disease.

Besides boosting strength and flexibility and helping you relax and feel good, yoga may actually ward off disease.

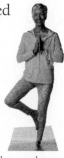

Multiple studies show that practicing yoga can reduce the need for pain medication in patients with arthritis, chronic back pain, and carpal-tunnel syndrome. A recent study out of the esteemed Cleveland Clinic shows that yoga is also good for bone health.

Other studies found that yoga reduced the number of angina attacks in patients with cardiovascular disease and that yoga may help control high blood pressure as effectively as some medications. Through its breathing exercises, yoga may also reduce the severity of chronic bronchitis and asthma.

Photo: gradyreese

The following exercises use a Pilates Circle, a steel ring 13 inches in diameter with foam-rubber handles, which you can purchase for less than $20…

571 Pilates Circle I: The big stretch.

Standing, raise the Pilates Circle over your head with both hands. Bend to one side slowly, to a count of eight. Hold for a count of eight. Rise slowly to a count of eight. Bend to the opposite side slowly, to a count of eight. Hold for a count of eight. Rise slowly to a count of eight.

Repeat 20 times, working up to 50 times. This exercise is great for strengthening your oblique muscles!

572 Pilates Circle II: Twist and shout.

Well, bend anyway. Standing, hold the Pilates Circle in front of you with both hands extended. Bend to one side slowly, to a count of eight. Hold for a count of eight. Bend to the opposite side slowly, to a count of eight. Hold for a count of eight. Rise slowly to a count of eight.

Repeat 20 times, working up to 50 times. This exercise is a wonderful waist-whittler!

573 Pilates Circle III: The big push.

You can do this exercise either standing or sitting. Hold the Pilates Circle by the handles, between your hands. Push forward as hard as you can, hold, then relax.

Repeat 20 times, working up to 50 times. This exercise is excellent for strengthening your biceps and can be a welcome change from lifting dumbbells.

574 Pilates Circle IV: Biceps pull.

Put one foam handle on your right shoulder. Hold the other handle in your right hand and pull down to a count of eight. Repeat 10 to 15 times. Then switch to your left shoulder and hand.

575 Pilates Circle V: Inner-thigh strengthener.

Stand and place the Pilates Circle with the foam handles between your thighs. Bring your thighs together and hold for a count of eight. Relax. Repeat 10 to 15 times.

This exercise is wonderful for shaping up the inner thighs, which tend to get flabby as we get older.

576 Don't resist resistance bands.

Resistance bands are simple rubber strips five to six inches wide that are available in different lengths or that your physical therapist often cuts off a roll and gives you for home exercises. They range in toughness from yellow (the easiest) to green to red to blue to black (the toughest). Most physical therapists use strips made by Thera-Band, which can be stretched or knotted. More expensive resistance bands are made of rubber tubing and have triangular handles at the ends, so they are less flexible.

577 Resistance band exercise I: Inner thigh I.

Many people have strong quad (front of the thigh) muscles, but much weaker medialis (inner thigh) muscles.

Strengthen these muscles even when you're lying on your back in bed by looping a knotted resistance band just under your knees. Bend your knees and place your feet flat. Spread your knees as far as they can go. Hold for a count of eight. Return to starting position. Repeat 16 times, then 20 times, then 30 times.

When this exercise becomes too easy, move up to the next-tougher resistance band.

578 Resistance band exercise II: Inner thigh II.

Standing, with your legs comfortably apart, loop a knotted resistance band just under your knees. Take a big step to your left until you can feel the pull in your inner thigh, then bring your right foot up to your left foot. Repeat 16 times. Then take a big step to your right and repeat.

When this exercise becomes too easy, move up to the next-tougher resistance band.

579 Resistance band exercise III: Upper and lower arms.

This exercise can be performed either sitting or standing, as long as your back is straight and you have enough room to extend your arms to the sides.

Hold one of the flat resistance bands in each fist or—for twice the workout—knot the resistance band and, with the knot in the center, hold the ends in each fist with your arms out in front of you. With your right hand steady, stretch the resistance band to the left. Return to the starting position, then repeat on the other side. Then stretch to both sides simultaneously.

Repeat this pattern 16 times, then 20 times, then 30 times.

When this exercise becomes too easy, move up to the next-tougher resistance band.

580 Laugh yourself to fitness.

Researchers at Stanford University have discovered that laughing for 30 seconds produces the same aerobic benefits as working out on a rowing machine for three minutes. What a delightful way to strengthen your abdominals! Bring on those classic Looney Tunes cartoons, *The Office*, *Family Guy*, *Seinfeld* and *The Big Bang Theory!*

581 Jump to it!

Jumping rope offers great aerobic benefits while it builds flexibility and coordination, and strengthens ankles and knees. One of its advantages is that it can be done in limited indoor space as well as outdoors. For extra fun, organize a jump-rope game with neighbors both older and younger than yourself. See how many of the schoolyard rope games and jump-rope rhymes you remember.

Get a game of Double Dutch going. You'll really glow! Pass these routines on to your kids and grandkids for wonderful multigenerational fun.

582 Draw that bow!

Have you ever yearned to play Robin Hood? Or Sheena, Queen of the Jungle? Grab a bow and arrow and yearn no more. Drawing a longbow is great exercise.

Although archery clubs abound, this can be a solo sport. All you need is a right- or left-hand longbow, a target, arrows, and an ample, protected space (i.e., no children or pets roaming about), like your backyard.

Pull the bowstring with your strong arm, and push the bow with your weak arm.

This means you'll need to practice other exercises with your weak arm, like standing one-handed push-ups against a wall or, if you're strong enough, one-handed push-ups on the floor.

583 Join in a pickup game.

Who says that playgrounds and dead end streets are only for kids? They can be ideal for casual games with loose rules, a chance for adults to put together softball or basketball games, to challenge their kids or the neighbors down the block.

If possible, try volleyball. If you can't locate or improvise a net, draw posts and a line representing the net in colored chalk. Volleyball is an excellent sport because players are in motion most of the time, combining lots of aerobics and stretching.

584 Exercise while you fly.

Long periods of sitting still can be very risky, especially for people who have circulatory or cardiovascular problems. The culprit is deep vein thrombosis (DVT), the formation of blood clots in the legs. If a clot breaks free and travels to the heart or the lungs, it can be fatal!

Here are some exercises you can do in your seat to increase circulation and decrease the risk of DVT...

585 Airborne I: Ankle circles.

Raise both feet off the floor. Rotate both of them simultaneously, making five circles toward the outside, then five toward the inside. Repeat this set five times. Try for once every hour.

586 Airborne II: Foot pumps.

Rock back on your heels, raising your toes as far as possible. Hold for a count of 10, then lower them to the floor. Now rock onto your toes, raising your heels as far as possible. Hold for a count of 10, then lower them to the floor. Repeat five times. Try for once every hour.

587 Airborne III: Shoulder rolls.

Place your arms on the armrests and move your shoulders in a circle from front to back 10 times. Repeat from back to front 10 times. Try for once every hour.

588 Airborne IV: Knee-to-chest stretches.

Lean forward slightly and clasp your hands around one knee. Pull it toward your chest slowly and hold for 15 seconds. Release. Switch to your other knee. Repeat five times. Try for once every hour.

589 Airborne V: Shoulder stretches.

Place your right hand on top of your left shoulder. Grasp your right elbow in your left hand and, keeping your right shoulder down, stretch your right shoulder gently toward your left side. Hold for 15 seconds. Switch sides and repeat. Do this set five times. Try for once every hour.

590 Airborne VI: Neck rolls.

Relax your head and shoulders. Stretch your neck toward your left shoulder, hold for five seconds, roll your head slowly toward your chest, then stretch toward your right shoulder. Hold for five seconds, then reverse, rolling your head from right to left. Repeat five times. Try for once every hour.

591 Exercise protects your brain.

Exercise really prevents the loss of brain tissue and the accompanying memory loss that starts in our 30s. MRI studies show that poorly controlled blood-glucose levels cause the brain's key memory center—the hippocampus—to shrink. But weight training, which builds muscle, regulates blood-glucose levels and helps prevent shrinkage of the brain tissue. Researchers believe that it can prevent or possibly even reverse memory loss.

592 Be reflective.

Play it safe when you exercise outdoors at dusk or night. Heighten your visibility to others by wearing reflective clothing, not clothing with reflective stripes, which reveal only a cartoonish outline of your shape.

593 Take fitness with you I: Choose hotels with exercise facilities.

Having a heavy travel schedule should not prevent your being able to work out. When you shop for a hotel, find out whether it has a gym, health club, pool—and whether there is a charge for using them. (If you get "sticker shock," find out if there is a running/walking trail near the hotel.)

594 Take fitness with you II: Use the passport program.

Check whether the health club you belong to—or are thinking of joining—is one of the thousands of clubs that participate in the International Health, Racquet & Sportclub Association (IHRSA) Passport Program, which lets you work out at any of the participating clubs while traveling in many countries around the world.

To use the Passport Program, log on to HealthClubs.com/passport, and follow the instructions. You'll be able to use any club more than 50 miles from your home club by paying a discounted guest fee. Call the guest club first to check hours, guest fee, and any restrictions.

595 Rev up your walking.

Perk up your walking workout by doing your usual warming up and stretching, walking briskly for 10 minutes, and then adding this quick little routine...

March in place for 30 seconds, lifting your knees high and swinging your arms. Walk briskly for one minute, then march in place again for 30 seconds. Continue walking briskly for 10 minutes, then add a second little routine...

Skip for 30 seconds, swinging your arms, walk briskly for one minute, then skip for 30 seconds.

Now continue your walking routine.

596 Invest in gripper-toe sandals.

Sandals that have ridges under your toes will improve your circulation and reduce the risk of diabetic neuropathy. As your toes grip the ridges, walking gives your legs an easy workout from your toes up to your thighs and glutes.

In addition, you will burn more calories than walking in ordinary shoes or sneakers.

597 Hoop it up!

Swinging a hula hoop around your middle can whittle your waistline and abs, trimming dangerous abdominal fat. It's a great cardiovascular workout, too.

Just make sure to rotate the hoop equally clockwise and counter-clockwise. We tend to favor our strong side, but you want to keep this workout evenly balanced.

598 Mind over mattress.

Drag your old mattress down to the basement or out to the backyard. Use it as a cushiony exercise mat or jump on it like a trampoline.

599 Be a Goody Two (pair of) Shoes.

Buy two identical-model pair of walking/exercise sneakers at the same time—ideally, at a two-for-one sale at the end of the season. Alternate wearing them. Airing them out in between wearings will reduce the risk of foot infection from bacteria—always a danger to individuals with diabetes.

600 Involve your employer I: Get a workplace exercise room.

Get together with your fellow employees to persuade your employer to turn unused or underused space into an exercise room. The cost to your employer can be as little as $5,000 tax-deductible business-expense dollars for a few exercise bicycles, a treadmill, a complete set of weights, and a large mirror. The benefits of this wellness initiative? Healthier employees, fewer sick days, and possibly even lowered health-insurance premiums.

601 Involve your employer II: Paying for your gym membership.

Many employers offer discounts or partial reimbursement for memberships in fitness clubs. Some employers will reimburse you $100 to $200 for every six-month period in which you visit the health club 60 times (two or three times a week). You'll be getting paid to keep fit!

602 Brighten up your treadmill space.

Most people who stop using their treadmills ditch them because they're boring. But as treadmills can be your key to fitness during the winter, it will pay off to make your treadmill environment more cheerful.

Try some of these ideas to brighten up your treadmill space and encourage its use: A brightly painted room or a poster or photo display on the wall, a vase with (artificial) flowers, plug-in fragrances, or a bowl of potpourri. Feeling lavish? Install a big-screen TV and/or a good music system. You'll never want to leave!

603 Easy walking lowers your blood pressure.

As people with diabetes are disproportionately susceptible to cardiovascular disease and stroke, discovering that any easy walking program lowers blood pressure enough to make an impact is a godsend.

According to a Japanese study from several years ago, walking only 20 minutes a day reduced the long-term risk of developing blood pressure in male study participants—enough to lower their overall risk of heart disease.

604 Do the one-mile workout without leaving home.

Bad weather? After dark? No problem. Put on some fast rock 'n' roll and do this snappy routine…

March in place	2 Minutes
Side steps, alternating starting foot	3
March in place	1
Knee lifts (march in place raising knees high)	3
March in place	1
Kicking out alternately, the higher the better	3
March in place	2
	15 Minutes
Distance	1 Mile

605 Make exercise a regular habit…especially if you're older.

Older people with diabetes need to exercise more frequently than younger ones. In a study published in the August 2003 issue of *Diabetes*, Mayo Clinic researchers found that exercise's effect of increasing the body's sensitivity to insulin may not last very long in older adults. In fact, after four or five days of not exercising, the ability of aerobic exercise to increase insulin sensitivity was still noticeable *only* in people younger than 40. Researchers concluded that you'll need to exercise at least every other day to maintain an ongoing insulin benefit if you are an older patient with diabetes.

606 Know that exercise combats metabolic syndrome.

"Metabolic syndrome" is defined as a cluster of common symptoms that increases the risk of diabetes and cardiovascular disease dramatically. *Diagnosis of metabolic syndrome requires at least three of these five identifying factors…*

•**Abdominal obesity** (a waist measuring over 40 inches for men, 35 inches for women)

•**Elevated triglycerides** (150 mg/dL or higher)

•**Low "good" HDL cholesterol** (less than 40 mg/dL in men, 50 mg/dL in women)

•**High blood pressure** (equal to or over 130 for systolic—top number—pressure, or equal to or over 85 for diastolic—bottom number—pressure)

•**Moderately elevated fasting blood glucose** (110 mg/dL-125 mg/dL, considered the threshold for diabetes)

Participants in the large U.S.-Canadian research study rode stationary bicycles for five months. At the end of the study, one-third of them originally diagnosed with metabolic syndrome no longer had the problem because they had reduced their waistlines, lowered their blood pressure, and improved their lab results. All of these positive changes indicate that exercise can eliminate metabolic syndrome in many people, thus reducing their risk of diabetes and heart disease.

607 Combine walking with hand weights.

You'll get much more of a workout if you add hand weights to your walking program. Start with one-pound weights and gradually work your way up to walking at four miles per hour with five-pound hand weights, which is equivalent to *running* at five miles per hour. Find weights that feel comfortable in both your hands by carrying them around the store for 10 minutes before you buy them. (But skip the weights if you have carpal-tunnel syndrome, arthritis in your hands, or shoulder problems.)

Photo: CHIARI_VFX

608 Walk backward, too.

Walking backward gives your hamstring and gluteus maximus muscles the workout that walking forward doesn't. So alternate one-minute intervals of walking backward with one minute of walking forward. Find a smooth, safe area, like a building hallway or track, if possible.

609 Half your walk, twice a day.

Exercising twice a day increases your metabolism and the calories you burn throughout the day. Do half your usual walk in the morning and half after dinner—or maybe five or 10 minutes more during one or both sessions.

610 Move it on up.

You may need to increase the iron you are pumping. Light weights will build muscle endurance, but heavier weights will whittle your shape and build solid muscle. Increase the weights slowly and decrease your repetitions. A gradual change from five-pound dumbbells to 10-pounders may be all you need.

611 Take shorter rests between sets.

Exercise experts recommend taking only 15 seconds to recover when you are lifting weights for strength training. That short interval gives you a little rest, but still keeps your heart rate up to burn more calories. (You'll lose that cardiovascular effect if you rest for even one or two minutes.)

612 Shadowbox.

Shadowboxing while you walk works your upper body and improves your posture. Use these moves for one minute at a time, or go freestyle...

Punch out straight in front of you at shoulder height. Then punch overhead. You can do all these punches with one fist and then change sides, or alternate between punches. Improvise!

613 Take a hike.

A walking vacation can combine days of serious exertion and cardiovascular benefits with exciting new experiences and the opportunity to make new friends.

Personal story: I went on a week's hike through the Welsh countryside as part of an organized walking tour covering about 60 miles. Because of the hard daily workout, not only was I able to skip my morning insulin every day, but I also lost five pounds despite eating very well.

614 Do longer walks on weekends.

Try to schedule at least a two-hour walk on pleasant weekends. Most cities and towns have beautiful parks or interesting historic districts. Many even have walking tours—check your weekend newspaper or the Internet.

For even more fun, turn this into a social event with friends or family, culminating in brunch or dinner.

615 Move laterally as well as forward.

To increase your workout and involve your inner and outer thigh muscles, add sideways motion to your walk. After a few minutes of walking, turn to the side, take 25 sideways steps wider than your shoulder width, turn, and do 25 more. Repeat as often as you like, changing sides.

616 Make your legs work harder.

Add lunges to your walk. Step forward on your right foot, keeping your knee over your heel. With your weight distributed evenly between both legs, lower your right thigh until it's parallel with the ground. Push off with your left foot to bring your feet together, and then lunge forward with your left foot. Alternate for 12 lunges with each leg, building up to 20. Repeat this pattern every three to five minutes during your walk.

617 Pick up the pace.

If you can, maintain your walking distance, but increase your speed. If you are presently walking a 20-minute mile, try for 18 minutes, then 15. Experts suggest increase your speed twice a week to achieve maximum results.

618 Jump for joy—and bone density.

As we get older, losing bone density is a problem, and osteoporosis is often the result—for men as well as for women.

Strengthen and protect your bones—and have fun!—by jumping on a trampoline five to 10 minutes at a time at least two or three times a week.

619 Make a rainy-day rockabilly riot!

It's raining or snowing, and nobody wants to take a walk in that—or drive to the mall to walk. So don't. Let The Killer (or one of his buddies) exercise you today. Draw the drapes and put on any music by Jerry Lee Lewis; there'll be a whole lot of shakin' going on. Carl Perkins, Chuck Berry, or any of their contemporaries can also get you up and moving. Johnny B. Goode!

620 Turn on a TV program that turns you off.

Everyone has a TV show they love to hate—either the political opinions are far from yours, or the sitcom dialogue is moronic, or the ugly contestant can't sing. Let that show inspire you to exertion. Whatever show or film gets your dander up, turn it on and turn it up.

Now give it the talking-to it deserves. Pace, flail your arms, talk back to the set, whatever loud activity gets you going. That dumb pundit won't have learned anything, but you'll feel better, physically and philosophically.

621 Bargain with that fast food with your feet.

The quickest path to an insatiable craving is that feeling of denial, so disarm that mechanism *now*. Tell yourself that you can have whichever fast food is calling your name so loudly—you just need to trade for it. Look through your calorie, carb, and fat list and "make room" for what you're craving, but first circle the restaurant twice before you go in.

Those few paces accomplish three goals: You'll have exercised a bit; your craving may have eased or even disappeared during your walk; and, at the very least, you can congratulate yourself for your sense and maturity—before you go ahead and indulge.

CHAPTER 6

Dealing with Depression and Stress

622 Learn to live with Murphy's Law.

Diabetes patients have a triple-barreled right to be angry and depressed. Diabetes is a chronic disease that can last more than 50 years. It requires constant attention and complex treatment, and can have some ugly consequences.

That's the first barrel.

The second barrel is the depression that can accompany diabetes, progressing from one stage of life to the next. Depression hits extra hard when you're an anxious teenager, a worried parent, or a middle-aged person coming to grips with aging.

The third barrel is Murphy's Law: If anything can possibly go wrong, it surely will.

You can eat exactly the same meal two days in a row. One day it will raise your blood glucose 20 points, the next day 100 points. Even endocrinologists don't always know why, and we get understandably frustrated that the specialists can't explain it to us.

That said, recognize the difference between short-term sadness that has a cause you can pinpoint, and longer-term true depression. After all, as American poet Delmore Schwartz pointed out, even paranoids have real enemies.

Still, if your blues last more than a week or two, contact your doctor or therapist.

623 Panic attack? No, it's dropping blood glucose.

Diabetes patients whose blood glucose swings from 160 to over 300—you know who you are, and please get help from your diabetes doctor!—can experience what they think is a panic attack when their blood glucose drops rapidly to between 80 and 100. They feel dizzy and shaky and think they're going to have a heart attack, or at least faint.

What to do? Check your blood glucose first. If it's 80 to 100, it's just a roller-coaster drop that's created your worrisome symptoms. Sit or lie down in a quiet place for 15 minutes and see if you feel better. If you don't, call 911 and get to an emergency room.

624 Great poetry for inner strength.

Find poetry about overcoming the vicissitudes of disease or aging that move you. *Some of my favorites…*

"Invictus" by William Ernest Henley

"Sailing to Byzantium" by W. B. Yeats

"Do Not Go Gentle Into That Good Night" by Dylan Thomas

"Rabbi Ben Ezra" by Robert Browning

I've memorized "Invictus"—it's short—and recite or read the others whenever I need special encouragement. You may find them useful at other times to get through rough patches.

625 Benefit from the canine connection.

I've often wondered how many dogs are named "Prozac."

Dogs are a marvelous antidepressant for many reasons:

• **Your dog loves you unconditionally and shows it often.**

• **Your dog will make sure that you get out at least twice a day.** This will give you fresh air, mild-to-vigorous exercise, and the opportunity to chat and socialize with other dog owners.

• **Your dog lets you be playful and silly, which will lift your spirits.**

626 Other pets help, too.

Although they may not provide the outdoor benefits, cats and other mammalian pets will cuddle and love you. You can play with them and be silly.

Fish are beautiful, and watching them is a great de-stresser. Birds are marvelous, and some species are extremely intelligent and can be trained to talk. (However, your African gray parrot may outlive you, so please make plans for him in your will.)

627 Find an older, happy role model.

My late aunt Rose, who died at the age of 98, is a perfect example. Although she was ill and housebound, she drew and painted, punned and wrote doggerel poetry. Her attitude? "If I wake up in the morning, it's going to be a good day." I often think of her and share her mantra with my friends.

628 Take a cue from Jimmy Durante.

Legendary nightclub entertainer, actor, and songwriter Jimmy Durante (1893–1980) was a master of the malapropism. The song he used to open his act can inspire all of us:

"You got to start off each day with a song
Even when things go wrong…"
Make it your mantra!

629 Buy a sassy T-shirt and wear it often.

One of my favorites has seven silhouettes depicting the rise of man from the apes, starting with what looks like a chimpanzee walking on its knuckles. While the center figure is striding along upright, the last figure is badly hunched over a computer, the caption: "Something, somewhere went terribly wrong."

Other smile provokers: T-shirts titled FEDERAL WITNESS PROTECTION PROGRAM in large capital letters, and anything with the Simpsons or Peanuts characters. My friend's favorite says, "IT SEEMED LIKE A GOOD IDEA AT THE TIME."

630 Child's play I: Blow bubbles I.

Think of how much fun you had blowing bubbles when you were a kid. Just the memory should make you smile.

Go to a toy or party store and buy bubble liquid and a wand, or a tube of plastic bubble goo. See what a huge bubble you can make!

If there is no toy or party store nearby and you get the urge, put some dishwashing liquid in a bowl, dip a pastry whisk in it, then blow at the whisk or shake or wave it to make a stream of bubbles.

631 Child's play II: Blow bubbles II.

The bubble gum of childhood now comes in a sugar-free version. You can order it from many sources on the Internet. Chew and pop that bubble gum and enjoy being a kid again!

632 Have fun with your enemies.

Put a picture of your most-hated politician, boss, or ex-love on a dartboard and throw darts at it.

633 Get your daily laughs.

Find political cartoons on the Internet. You'll find funny, satirical ones regardless of your opinion. A good site is EditorialCartoonists.com, the website of the Association of American Editorial Cartoonists. Or find funny video sites, like Funny or Die, or search favorite clips on YouTube.

634 Get out and garden...

Gardening lets you connect with the natural world and create and nurture beauty. You don't need a large plot of land to grow flowers or herbs; even window boxes have enough space. Or grow indoor plants like African violets or cacti and other succulents, or start a sweet potato vine in a jar of water.

Many neighborhoods have community gardens. They are wonderful places to improve your gardening skills and to make new friends.

635 ...Or visit one...

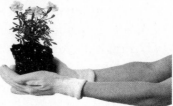

Nearly every large city boasts at least one magnificent botanical garden. Turn your visit into a mini-vacation; arrive early and stay late. Take a picnic lunch and a blanket, a camera and a notebook, a sketchbook, and crayons or pastels. Stroll along the paths and let your mind drift into neutral. Enjoy all the beauty!

Photo: EHStock

Or visit a friend's garden. Offer to help weed or rake to ensure your welcome.

636 ...Or be an armchair gardener.

If the preceding tips are inconvenient, be an armchair gardener. Borrow gardening books from the library. Get seed and plant catalogs. Research specific gardening issues on the Internet.

Are you more ambitious? More creative? Plan your dream garden on graph paper, or on your computer, or sketch it. One day you may achieve it!

637 Volunteer at an animal shelter.

Any kind of volunteering is good for your soul. When you volunteer at an animal shelter, you usually feed and water the animals, play with them and pet them, getting them used to being touched by loving hands.

Walking shelter dogs is a pleasant chore. You get to socialize with several dogs at every visit and also get a lot of exercise you don't have to think about.

638 Train your dog to be a therapy pet.

Calm, friendly, well-behaved dogs between the ages of one and 10 make ideal therapy pets. After evaluation and a training session, you and your dog will be visiting nursing homes, hospitals, and rehabilitation centers, improving the quality of life for institutionalized patients. Dogs provide excellent rehab opportunities. Patients who refuse physical therapy will gladly throw a ball for your dog, or walk him or her. Autistic or withdrawn patients are happy to talk to your dog. And your volunteering will make you glow!

639 Get enough sleep.

Sleep deprivation is a major cause of depression. Most adults need eight to nine hours of sleep a night; a few need as little as seven or as much as 10. Without naps, very few people are alert and happy on only five or six hours of sleep.

Catching up on your sleep on weekends doesn't work very well. You really need to get a good night's sleep every night. Try going to bed a half hour earlier for a week, then an hour earlier. See if you're not more cheerful!

640 Don't let SAD sadden you.

SAD (seasonal affective disorder) is the medical term for the winter blues, the depression that occurs because the days are shorter and often bleak and gloomy.

Take advantage of every sunny day to get out and walk for at least a half hour. But if the sun is strong, use a sunscreen or sunblock and wear sunglasses and a hat.

If you live in an area with few sunny winter days, you might want to purchase lightbulbs that are designed to mimic sunlight. And if that doesn't lift your spirits, talk to your doctor about trying a mild antidepressant for the Thanksgiving-Easter period.

641 Start building your castle.

Borrow your children's Lego blocks or Lincoln Logs, or buy them used in thrift shops, flea markets, or yard sales.

Get down on the floor and have fun!

642 You are not a number.

Do you remember *The Prisoner*, the groundbreaking TV fantasy series of the late 1960s, in which Patrick McGoohan (Number 6) frequently cries out, "I am not a number, I am a free man!"

You, too, are not a number. You are much more than your blood-glucose number or your glycohemoglobin A1C number, which may be high and which may depress you. You, too, are a free person, and you are free to improve your numbers.

Don 't let the "numbers game" get you down. You are a whole person, a unique individual.

643 Play a kazoo.

The kazoo is an inexpensive musical instrument that can be learned very quickly and takes no talent whatsoever to play well. Maybe that's why it's been around since 1884, according to Webster's dictionary. All you have to do to make music is hum through the tube.

If you get the urge and there's no toy store near you, just put a tissue paper over a comb and start humming.

644 Apply a "cockamamie."

Even the name makes me smile. It's a corruption of the word "decalcomania," which we New York kids had probably never heard and couldn't have pronounced. It's a temporary tattoo, which you can buy in toy and cosmetics stores.

Applying them now can bring us back to childhood, or can be used for a devil-may-care or erotic gesture. Put them where the world can see them, or just a special someone. They'll last for about five days, but you can wash them off earlier if you get tired of them. My favorites are Harley-Davidson logos—all the swashbuckling and bravado, none of the pain or permanence.

645 Take a mini-cruise.

There's something wonderfully soothing about being on the water—even for just an hour or two. Most cities near lakes, rivers, or oceans offer a variety of inexpensive water trips, sometimes combined with dinner, music, a historical tour, or even whale watching. Even an off-hour commuter ferry can be fun.

When you return, you'll probably feel refreshed and better able to focus.

646 Read biographies for inspiration.

People who have accomplished great things or made momentous discoveries—often in the face of poverty or disability—can inspire us to overcome our own problems that we think are insurmountable.

Read the lives of the great geniuses—Ludwig van Beethoven or Thomas Alva Edison—whose creative output was astonishing, despite their deafness. Of Winston Churchill, who battled his "black dogs" of depression as well as World War II's Axis Powers. More recently sainted Mother Teresa, who fought poverty and disease as well as the rigid Roman Catholic establishment.

Although not a biography in the strictest sense, the letters of Vincent van Gogh—mostly to his brother Theo—are extremely revealing and inspirational.

647 Collect a library of funniest films.

You might want to start at the American Film Institute's website, which features the 100 Funniest, or list your own favorites and build your collection. Some personal favorites: *The Producers*, Marx Brothers' outrageous classics *Duck Soup* and *A Night at the Opera*, the screwball comedy *Bringing Up Baby*, W. C. Fields's last starring film, *Never Give a Sucker an Even Break*, featuring the world's most hysterical car chase, and the Christopher Guest mockumentaries, *Best in Show* and *Waiting for Guffman*.

Relax for a couple of hours, download one of these classics, and convulse with laughter.

648 Go back to school.

Increase your knowledge or learn a new skill at your local community college, library, or YMCA. Hundreds of courses are available every semester. Learn a foreign language, develop your creative skills, or study a subject you always wanted to when you were younger.

649 Tea can get you through.

The British standby, "a nice hot cup of tea" has seen millions through all kinds of adversity. It may be the calming liquid, but it's also probably the ritual. Late in the afternoon, stop everything and break for tea. When you return to work or your daily chores, everything seems clearer, more manageable.

650 Vary your daily routine.

Do you always walk or drive along the same route? Do your laundry on the same day of the week? Maybe that's what's getting you down.

Change your daily routine a little. Take a different route to or from work. Save your chores for a different day of the week. Better yet, list how many aren't really necessary—and don't do them until next week or next month.

651 Don't be your own worst enemy.

Ditch your unreasonable expectations for yourself. They are a major cause of chronic depression, which makes your diabetes worse and more difficult to control.

Cut yourself some slack. Be as forgiving with yourself as you are with your best friends.

Make two lists: "Five Things I Like About Myself" and "Five Things I'm Proud Of." Keep them in your wallet and look at them frequently.

652 Smile at your neighbors.

The physical act of smiling is a powerful antidepressant.

Smile at neighborhood children and at people walking their dogs. Engage them in conversation. You will feel less isolated, and you may learn new things.

653 Buy yourself flowers.

Flowers are an inexpensive indulgence. In Manhattan, a little judicious shopping will get you a dozen roses for only $15.

Two dozen roses are a lavish gift from you to you in appreciation of your existence. Take the time to arrange them gloriously in one or more vases. Steal one rose for your night table, another for your bathroom. Enjoy all their natural beauty!

654 Learn from the Serenity Prayer.

The great American liberal theologian Reinhold Niebuhr's "Serenity Prayer" has been a mantra for millions of people who try to live by these simple, profound words: "God grant me the serenity to accept the things I cannot change, courage to change the things I can, and the wisdom to know the difference."

Focus on the "serenity" and "courage," and your mood will lift.

655 Find beauty with a kaleidoscope.

A kaleidoscope isn't just a kid's toy. You can use it to facilitate meditation and find your "quiet place." Rotate the collar, and suddenly the brightly colored bits of glass turn into the mesmerizing rose windows of Notre-Dame Cathedral in Paris.

A teleidoscope works the same way, but uses just a lens and mirrors that reflect and multiply whatever you point it at, much the way a fly's eye works, so that you will see real objects broken into myriad planes, making fascinating patterns.

656 Rosemary can rev you up.

Hamlet's Ophelia may have shortchanged rosemary; she praised it for "remembrance." The herb's aroma fights fatigue by triggering the release of *norepinephrine*, a brain chemical that lifts energy levels. It also increases beta brainwaves, which are associated with alertness.

657 **Bright colors lift your spirits.**

Depression feeds on black clothing. Think of all the negative figures of speech associated with "black," versus "being in the pink."

But don't dump your basic black. Perk up your wardrobe, ladies, with bright-colored scarves and jewelry; men, with bright or cartoon-motif ties.

You'll feel better when you look into the mirror, and other people will respond to you more positively.

658 **Wear fragrance.**

Fragrance has the power to banish the blues. When you wear cologne or aftershave, you automatically feel more attractive to yourself and to the rest of the world.

You can intensify this feeling by wearing an old favorite that you wore years ago.

Here's why it works: Scent-evoked nostalgia is so strong because there is a direct connection between the olfactory bulb at the top of your nasal cavity and your hypothalamus, your brain's memory center. When you wear a favorite old fragrance, you can remember all the happy, intense emotions you experienced when you wore it in the past.

659 **Follow the lure of lemons.**

Did you ever wonder why furniture polish and other products contain lemon oil? Lemon smells good, and it's also energizing. Experts say that the scent of lemon contains *turpine*, a biochemical that increases alertness by stimulating the trigeminal nerve, the principal sensory nerve of your face.

Enjoy fresh lemon peel in potpourri. Mix equal parts of lemon peel with chopped lemongrass, dried lemon verbena leaves, or rosemary. When your potpourri loses its fragrance, wrap it in cheesecloth and put it into your bath to release the last of its scent.

660 **Heads up!**

Actors know how to create character through posture and physical movement. They express confidence and alertness with an upright head and forceful physical actions. They express depression with a hangdog posture and hesitant movements.

Learn from actors. When you keep your head up and move confidently, your movements will make you feel less depressed.

661 Break the bad posture chain.

Poor posture leads to migraine and back pain, and pain is a major cause of depression. Spending hours at a time hunched over a keyboard can cause what orthopedists call "postural syndrome" or "postural derangement," which can trigger neck, shoulder, and back pain, and the resultant depression. It's hard to be happy when you're hurting.

Breaking this chain is not difficult, but it requires developing and practicing new habits. Start by taking 30-second breaks from the computer to stand up, stretch, take a few deep breaths, and stand very straight, like the military "attention" posture.

More structured exercise, like yoga or Pilates, will help you achieve pain-free good posture, too.

662 Are breathing problems causing your depression?

It's hard to be happy when you're having trouble breathing. If you're often short of breath, it could be allergies, asthma, emphysema, or something else.

Best bet: See a pulmonologist (lung specialist). When your breathing problem is diagnosed and treated, your depression will likely improve.

663 Find a mantra.

Mantras—words or phrases repeated as invocations or incantations—have de-stressed millions of people and helped them focus over the centuries. *One or more of these may work for you…*

"Om"

"Peace"

"I believe"

My favorite is the Biblical "And it came to pass," because of its eternal wisdom and perspective. The Bible never says, "And it came to stay."

664 Read a sacred work.

Holy books have consoled us and strengthened our faith for thousands of years through their enduring wisdom.

Read the Old or New Testament, the Koran, the Upanishads, or the Bhagavad Gita. Or, if you do not feel traditionally religious, you may feel more comfortable—and comforted—with the *Book of Psalms* or *Meditations* by Marcus Aurelius.

665 Attend religious services.

These, too, can banish depression and stress and lift your spirits.

Being part of a community of worship also strengthens the feeling that you are not alone in this world.

666 Count your blessings.

When you focus on your blessings, you realize that your cup is half-full, not half-empty.

Be thankful for family and friends, for your job or profession, for your home, for all the things that you enjoy. Write them down—you'll be surprised how many you can list!

667 Follow your bliss.

Mythologist and folklorist Joseph Campbell, subject of the Bill Moyers PBS series *The Power of Myth,* coined the phrase "Follow your bliss" to describe the burning need that individuals and societies have to identify and pursue what they feel passionate about.

Following your bliss leaves little room for depression and stress. Passion and excitement drive them out and create an environment for happiness and joy.

668 Widen your circle of friends.

One of the consequences of modern life is an extremely mobile population. Nowhere is it more visible—or more psychologically damaging—than in how our friendships must change. *Personal story*: Several years ago, my two best friends moved from my Manhattan neighborhood—one to Long Island, the other to Orlando. As a result, I see them about once a year, instead of once or twice a week.

Widening your circle of friends protects you from suddenly losing your best friends. There's safety in numbers!

669 Light candles.

Most of the world's great faiths light candles in their religious rituals. They symbolize light in the darkness, hope in a world of uncertainty.

You, too, can benefit from the symbolism of candles. You can use them to focus when you are praying or meditating. Or they can banish the winter blues. They also create a festive atmosphere, and that, too, can generate happiness.

670 Join a support group.

Support groups give you *many* brains solving problems and sharing experiences. And their discussions often spark creative new ideas. They are definitely worth trying. And if your first support group isn't helpful or has some obnoxious participants, try other groups.

You can Google "support groups" for diabetes, depression, and many other topics.

671 Use message boards.

Message boards offer all the advantages of support groups, plus two more big ones: Anonymity and the flexibility of visiting and contributing only when it is convenient for you.

Here too, you can Google "message boards" for diabetes, depression, and many other topics.

672 Do three good deeds a day.

This should be a desirable goal, not an inflexible rule. Good deeds take you out of yourself and can help you forget your diabetes for a while.

Your good deed can be a little thing, like holding a door or an elevator for someone with a lot of packages, or phoning a friend or neighbor just to touch base. Or it can be something major, like visiting a shut-in or a hospitalized friend, or helping a neighbor who has a toddler and an infant.

Whatever good deed you do, you will feel better as a result.

673 Find your quiet place.

Your quiet place can remove your stress. It can be real—a favorite armchair or the bathtub…or mental (Tahiti)…or even imaginary (Middle Earth).

What counts is that you can send your body or your mind to that magical center to drift and relax. You will return refreshed and destressed.

Note: If your imagination could use some inspiration, try guided-imagery recordings (something else you can easily find with a Google search).

674 Volunteer.

Every community needs volunteers, and volunteering is a more structured way of doing three good deeds a day.

Most cities and towns can use hundreds of volunteers, so your choices can be wide. Check with your mayor's office or your city's website for options.

675 Treat every day as a gift.

Since our national disaster of September 11, 2001, most of us are mindful that life is uncertain. Make the most of each day. Regard it as a golden opportunity to do something special, to be someone special.

676 Focus on the present and the future.

No one can change the past. You can learn from it but you can't change it, and it's self-destructive to obsess over it and to play the "If only I had/If only I hadn't" game. And self-destructive behavior creates stress and leads to depression.

Instead, focus on the present and the future. What can you do today, this week, this year to improve your health and your life?

677 Try meditation before medication…

Western medicine is pill-oriented. Antidepressants are a billion-dollar industry. But many people with diabetes don't like taking another batch of pills on top of the diabetes, cholesterol-lowering, and stroke-prevention medications they are already taking.

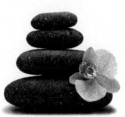

Try meditation first. Find your quiet place and let your mind wander. Experiment and see which technique

Photo: Ljupco

works for you. If you feel less depressed after a couple of weeks, you may not need antidepressant medication at all.

678 …But medication does not mean failure.

Because every person has a unique brain biochemistry, antidepressant medication may turn out to be the best solution. If pills work better for you than meditation or other therapies, do not regard it as a personal failure—that's just the way your brain is wired.

Make your goal, "Whatever works best for me."

679 Watsu may work for you.

What is Watsu? A trademarked abbreviation of "water shiatsu," a therapy that combines therapeutic massage with water's healing properties.

Developed at a California hot-springs retreat in the 1980s, Watsu is now practiced by many massage therapists. Clients start in a pool of 98-degree water, the same as your body temperature. The warm water and gravity-reduced environment induce deep relaxation and help your spine and tense muscles let go.

Massage is the second part of the session. Many clients who experience Watsu find that it drives out feelings of tension, rage, depression, and stress.

680 Dress for success.

Any form of discomfort can induce or add to already-existing stress. Avoid tight, overly restrictive clothing or clothing that is too loose or too baggy.

Clothing that fits comfortably and is neither too warm or too lightweight will make you feel better, look better, and be more relaxed. If your workplace environment differs markedly from the outdoors, dress in layers so that you'll always feel comfortable, indoors and out.

681 It's stress, buster.

Your job is often a cause of stress. Sometimes taking a break and walking around the block will do wonders to alleviate your stress. Any mild exercise will often do the trick, but Type A people have to remember that life is not a contest, and not to create more stress by overdoing it.

682 Use a touchstone to beat workplace stress.

A touchstone, in this context, is an object that you pass by frequently during your workday. Your personal touchstone might be a plant, a photograph, or even the water cooler. After you choose your touchstone, put your hand on it whenever you pass it and keep it there for a couple of seconds. Let this gesture remind you to breathe more deeply, to focus, to take a short break. This technique, called "grounding" or "anchoring," helps to reduce stress.

683 Connect with your special talisman.

This object, believed to contain magical properties to provide good luck or protection from evil or harm, can be as old-fashioned as a rabbit's foot or as simple as a "lucky coin."

My talisman is a paperweight inscribed with the jokey adolescent Latin "*Illegitimus non carborundum est*," which translates "Don't let the b*st*rds grind you down." If I want to meditate, I just stare at it and burst out laughing. It's a great antidepressant!

684 Always have a "Plan B."

It's a fact of life that few things go according to schedule. Curveballs abound.

If you are not flexible and don't have an alternative plan, you're going to get stressed out. Having and following a "Plan B" will prevent that from happening.

685 Silent nights lower stress.

Living in a noisy neighborhood can raise your stress level, especially when you sleep. As a survival mechanism, most people's auditory systems are still working when they are asleep, on the alert for sounds that signify danger. A noisy environment increases the production of stress hormones.

Why is that important? Excessive blood levels of the stress hormone cortisol have been linked to an increased risk of aging and disease, especially insulin resistance and cardiovascular disease.

What can you do about it? The easiest solution is to wear earplugs. If they don't work for you, try a TV or radio station that plays soft music uninterrupted by commercials or a machine that plays a continuous tape of a waterfall to drown out the noise.

686 Statins may reduce depression risk.

Statin drugs like Lescol (*fluvastatin*), Lipitor (*atorvastatin*), Mevacor (*lovastatin*), Pravachol (*pravastatin*), and Zocor (*simvastatin*) are used to lower cholesterol and are being prescribed for diabetes patients even if their cholesterol is low or normal because statins can cut the risk of cardiovascular disease and stroke in diabetic patients by about one-third.

Now it appears that statins may also lower depression risk when they are used continuously for many years. After average use of four years, patients on statin therapy had a 30% to 40% reduced risk of depression and lower levels of hostility and anxiety. Every additional year of statin therapy lowered these risks even more.

A 2015 study by SW. Kim and colleagues in *Translational Psychiatry* suggested that statins can improve depression independent of antidepressant use, but combining statins with antidepressants may have an even more powerful effect on depression.

687 Nobody's perfect—and that means you.

Insisting on being perfect, especially in minor things, is a recipe for major stress and for the depression that results because you're not perfect. No one is!

Give yourself permission to put most issues and tasks into the "not really all that important" category. Remember that the best baseball players in history struck out more than 70% of the time.

688 Destroy ANTs (automatic negative thoughts).

This clever acronym was coined by brain-disorder expert and best-selling author of *Change Your Brain, Change Your Life*, Daniel G. Amen, MD.

Because these negative thoughts are automatic, you have to interrupt them so that your poor, bedeviled brain doesn't whirl around and around like a hamster wheel.

How do you do this? Find some self-talk that works for you.

Here are some useful phrases: "Oh, come on! You don't really believe this!" Or "Yeah, and there's a bridge I'd like to sell you," a line familiar to most New Yorkers.

689 Frequent fatigue? Keep a log.

As frequent fatigue is often a source of stress or depression, keeping a daily log for at least a month can help you and your doctors identify the cause.

Does your fatigue occur at the same time just about every day? What events trigger it? How long does it last? The more detailed the history you can give your doctors, the easier it will be to diagnose your frequent fatigue and treat it.

690 Fight depression I: Stay fit.

Physical fitness helps the body to help the mind. Feeling better and having better flexibility, strength, and endurance and more energy will go a long way to make your outlook more positive, more confident, more able to cope with everyday problems and hassles. *Mens sana in corpore sano!* (A healthy mind in a healthy body.)

691 Fight depression II: Stay active.

Maintaining a routine will alleviate boredom, which feeds depression. Having other things to think about, having things to look forward to every day, will help you avoid aimlessness, which is one of depression's greatest allies.

692 Fight depression III: Stay focused.

The mental aspect of fighting aimlessness is not letting your attitude slide any more than your physical activity does. Live your life each day and keep your goals in front of you, even if it's only a trip to the local store. Don't talk yourself into procrastination.

If you have problems staying focused, make a "to-do" list the night before. Number your tasks and check them off as you complete them.

693 Fight depression IV: Stay comfortable.

Physical discomfort magnifies depression. Almost all brainwashing begins with physical discomfort, not pain. Make sure your living space is warm or cool enough, that your clothes aren't too restricting, that your shoes don't pinch, that you have enough of the right food to eat. Take care of your physical body, and that will help take care of your mind.

694 Create a pleasurable wake-up ritual.

Enjoyable early-morning rituals will destress you and help you face the day.

Do your windows face east? Sleep with your window shades up and let the sun wake you.

Awake to the aroma of freshly brewed coffee by programming your coffee-maker the night before. Almost as good as having a butler, isn't it?

Set your clock radio to your favorite music station—maybe even a little early, so that you can hit the snooze button and still be on time.

695 Unwind after work.

When you get home, take a five- or 10-minute break. Kick back, take off your shoes, and put your feet up on the nearest piece of furniture. Take a few deep breaths and let them out slowly.

That short break is all it takes. Now you can face the rest of your evening without carrying over any workplace stress.

696 Getting ready the night before eliminates morning stress.

After dinner, listen to the weather forecast, then lay out tomorrow's clothes. Are they clean and pressed? No buttons missing? No open seams? Shoes polished?

Next, pack your briefcase or backpack with everything you'll need and get tomorrow's lunch ready if you're brown bagging it.

Tomorrow morning should go smoothly, with no little unwelcome surprises. And you'll have removed a major source of stress.

697 High blood glucose increases stress by affecting your thinking.

You know that low blood glucose (hypoglycemia) clouds your thinking and raises your anxiety and stress level because your mind just isn't working well. But did you realize that high blood sugars alter your thinking almost as much? Even short-term spikes in blood glucose can sap your mental sharpness, verbal ability, and mathematical skills.

Avoid stress by keeping your blood-glucose levels as even as possible.

698 Connect with nature.

Take a few minutes to look—*really* look—at a flower, a tree, a bird, a squirrel. Notice how the sunlight strikes the buds or shines through the translucent petals or filters through the leaves.

If you are observing a bird or a squirrel, stay very still and they may approach you out of curiosity. (Or lure them with sunflower seeds. Just be aware that one bird may turn into a flock.)

In connecting with nature during this brief, quiet interval, you will be letting your stress flow out of your mind and your body.

699   A catnap can be your catnip.

Even the briefest nap can revive you, lower your stress, and lift your spirits. The great Winston Churchill attributed his clear strategic thinking, energy, and boundless optimism during the crises of World War II to his frequent daily catnaps.

Let catnaps work for you, too.

700   Reading drives out depression.

Listen to the words of essayist and philosopher Michel de Montaigne (1533–1592), arguably the greatest mind of the French Renaissance, who sometimes got depressed, too:

"When I am attacked by gloomy thoughts, nothing helps me so much as running to my books. They quickly absorb me and banish the clouds from my mind."

Don't those words strike a chord in us five centuries later?

701   Make bill paying less onerous.

Let's face it: No one enjoys paying bills. But using illustrated checks can make the chore less burdensome.

You can choose from more than 100 designs, including comic-strip characters, animals, flowers and landscapes, and Bible verses.

My personal favorite: Vintage Harley-Davidson motorcycles.

Note: I am strongly against banking online. There are too many opportunities to get hacked.

702   Swap hated chores with a neighbor…

Chances are you don't hate the same chores equally, so trade off with a neighbor.

One of you cleans both your ovens, the other washes and waxes both your floors. Before Thanksgiving, one of you hand washes both precious china and crystal collections, the other polishes your silver and your friend's.

Isn't this a less stressful way of handling the chores you hate?

703 …Or hire a neighborhood kid to do them.

Most kids need more spending money than their allowances give them, and they are willing to work for it.

Benefit from their energy and strong muscles by hiring them to do the chores you hate the most.

704 Walk on air.

One of the fastest, easiest, and least expensive treatments for depression and stress may be a pair of gel insoles for your shoes or sneakers. They make walking easier and put a spring in your step. And when your feet are happy…

705 Stay out of debt.

Financial problems can worry us day and night, draining our mental and physical energy. That's a prime recipe for depression and stress.

Creating a realistic monthly and yearly budget is a crucial first step. Include categories for savings and leisure. Careful planning will help you avoid living from paycheck to paycheck.

706 Cuddle with that special someone.

Act like a teenager again and cuddle on the living room couch. Express your loving feelings! Share your dreams and plans.

707 Massage your neck and scalp.

Do you feel a tension headache coming on? Defuse that stress by massaging your neck and scalp.

Start at the back of your neck with the fingertips of one or both hands. Move your fingertips in small circles, using as much pressure as you're comfortable with. Then move your fingertips in small circles over your scalp. This will increase the flow of blood to the area and minimize the likelihood of a full-blown tension headache.

708 Practice random acts of kindness.

The gospel "Practice random acts of kindness and senseless acts of beauty" was created by Ann Herbert in 1982 and has since spread around the world.

Many cities celebrate a Random Acts of Kindness Week during the second week of February with special projects and programs.

For suggestions as to what you can do on this special week or even every day, log on to the Random Acts of Kindness Foundation website, RandomActs ofKindness.org.

709 Solve puzzles.

Stimulating your brain is a wonderful antidepressant.

Puzzles are ideal because many types are so portable. All you need for them is a pencil or a pen. You can pick them up whenever you have a few minutes, then put them down again. Try crosswords, acrostics, or jumbled words. You can find many apps on your phone.

When you have more time and space—like a rainy weekend—you may want to try solving chess problems or doing a jigsaw puzzle.

710 Work smarter, not harder.

Start every task by thinking about it for a few moments. Is there a better or easier way to do this job? Saving time and effort will make you feel so much better!

711 Lighten your to-do list.

Many of us make a "to-do" list every morning or the night before, if we're extremely organized. Then we check off every item on the list after we do it.

That's very organized—but honestly, now, are all of these tasks absolutely necessary? If you had the time to do only five or 10 of them, would this particular task still be on your list? Could you eliminate it? Postpone it? Combine it with another task?

Or, if you prefer the words of the visionary business consultant and philosopher Peter F. Drucker, "There is nothing so useless as doing efficiently that which should not be done at all."

Now that you have a management expert's permission, do something happy and relaxing with the time you've freed up.

712 Give yourself a spa day.

Don't wait for your partner or your kids to give you a gift certificate. And it won't be necessary to empty the piggy bank. This is something you can do for yourself at home for less than $10 to $15.

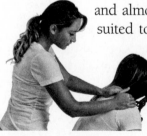

Start with a facial—guys, too. Use a grainy soap like oatmeal and almond and a loofah sponge. Follow up with a masque suited to your skin type. Spread it over your face, avoiding your eyes, and remove it with a warm, wet washcloth. Then apply a moisturizer. You'll look and feel so much younger! Just peek in the mirror.

Now take a long soak in the bathtub. Put a cup of oatmeal into a cut-off pantyhose leg. Save the orange peel from breakfast, cut it into small pieces to

Photo: Justin Horrocks

182

release the fragrant oils, put the pieces into the pantyhose leg, knot it, and toss it into the tub. Fill the tub with water as hot as you can stand it and get in with a magazine or paperback. Stay in for at least 20 minutes and just relax.

After you get out of the tub, moisturize. Then put on sweats or comfortable old clothes. Give yourself a manicure and pedicure, or just slather cream on your hands and feet and put on cotton gloves and socks for an hour. Put your feet up.

Spend the rest of the day just relaxing.

713 Join a book club.

Participate in a book club with a small group of people who read the sort of books you enjoy, whether it be classic literature, modern fiction, fantasy and science fiction, travel essays, poetry, history, or biographies. Reading a book to discuss it is a very different experience from reading a book on your own; take notes while you read so that you can discuss the book more intelligently.

Some people like to join book clubs where a kind of book they don't usually read is discussed, so as to open new genres for their enjoyment.

Most book clubs read a book a week or every two weeks. If you can't form a book club from among your friends, most independent bookstores as well as the large chains offer congenial groups.

714 Music live or online.

Let live music lift your spirits. See local musical groups perform in cafes and bookstores—almost always for free. Splurge on tickets for the opera or symphony.

If you're an online type, take advantage of the wonderful songs on YouTube or listen to your favorite genre using the smartphone apps Spotify or iHeartRadio. Even if you can't afford to buy a lot, sometimes listening to eight bars of that oldie you remember from years ago is enough to lift your spirits.

715 Keep a journal.

Write regularly in a journal. It can help center you and organize thought processes that may seem chaotic at the time.

716 Delight in online comic strips.

You can get them online through many sources. Out of the 50 or 60, you'll probably find a dozen favorites. It's nice to have something to laugh at every day!

My favorites: Cathy, Dilbert, and *The Wizard of Id.*

717 Try dancing...

Take dance lessons. Even if you don't care much about dancing, the lessons can be wonderful for putting you in touch with your body, making you feel more in tune with yourself and more graceful at a time when you might feel angry at your body for letting you down.

718 ...or yoga.

Yoga classes can often provide the same benefits as dance classes, with the added advantage that many will teach you how to meditate and center yourself. Choose a class at a yoga center, not one given by a gym, unless you want to use the class merely for exercise.

719 Take a little risk.

No, not skydiving without a parachute or riding your bike without a helmet, but doing something that's a little bit outside your comfort zone.

Maybe it's just buying a lottery ticket once in a while, or taking a three- or five-mile hike if you're not sure you can run a marathon.

What counts is opening yourself to new experiences.

720 Look up an old friend.

You lost touch years ago; you may not even remember exactly when or why. Perhaps one of you moved or changed jobs.

Make today the day to reconnect. Grab your old Rolodex or address book and pick up your phone! Or connect on Facebook or LinkedIn.

721 Start a kaffeeklatsch.

Get together with some friends, neighbors, or coworkers once a week for coffee. No agendas, just socialize and enjoy your time together. (My Australian friend Len, who has been doing this for close to 50 years calls this weekly event his "Blokes' Breakfast.")

722 Boys'/girls' night out.

It doesn't have to be at night, either. Just a group of guys or gals having fun together.

723 Groom your pet.

Spend five or 10 minutes a day combing or brushing your pet. Use long, slow strokes. Look into his/her eyes and have a one-sided conversation.

He will love the undivided attention. And you will feel better and more relaxed, too.

724 Rent a three-handkerchief movie.

Sometimes you need a good cry when you feel depressed or stressed. The best way to release your feelings is to watch the kind of film that legendary directors called a "three-handkerchief movie."

Here are some personal recommendations to start you off...

The Elephant Man
Equus
I'll Cry Tomorrow
It's a Wonderful Life
On Golden Pond
Love Story
Titanic

725 The joy of fingerpainting.

You don't have to be able to draw to take advantage of the joyful experience of fingerpainting.

This is your opportunity to be spontaneous—even messy. To connect with your Inner Child. Doesn't it feel wonderful?

Save your best efforts. Post them on the refrigerator or even frame and hang them.

Added bonus: You'll smile as you walk by them.

726 Be camera ready.

Spend a morning or afternoon with your camera in a park or historic district of your town. For this little adventure, buy a disposable camera at your local drugstore for around $10. Heaven forbid you should drop your phone at that beautiful lakeside view. No loss if you drop your disposable.

Pretend that you are a photography student on assignment to take the most unusual pictures, and don't go home until you finish the roll.

Won't you be surprised when you see the developed pictures!

727 Rekindle 100 strokes.

Ladies, did your grandmother train you to brush your hair 100 strokes every night?

This old-fashioned beauty ritual requires bending at the waist and dropping your head. This move alone will relax your neck muscles and increase the flow of blood to your head and neck.

Then, with a natural-bristle hairbrush, brush your hair from the roots to the ends, following each brush stroke with a similar stroke from the palm of your opposite hand. This motion counts as one stroke.

Concentrating on the brushing and the counting will free your mind. And not only will this ritual de-stress you, but your hair will become much glossier and your complexion will glow more.

728 Breathe easy.

A great deal of our daily stress is both the cause and the result of shallow breathing. We are stressed, so we don't breathe deeply. And because we are not taking in enough oxygen, our bodies are not functioning at their best, and we become stressed.

Break this vicious circle. At least once every hour, breathe as deeply as you can. Feel your lungs filling up, all the way from the bottom to the top. Take at least five breaths this way every hour.

At the end of a week, ask yourself whether you've felt less stressed. The answer will likely be yes.

729 Through a child's eyes.

Seeing the world through a child's eyes can reawaken your sense of wonder. To a young child, even the most mundane events and experiences are novel. If you do not have small children or grandchildren of your own, borrow a neighbor's child for an hour or two and see what both of you can discover!

730 Play tourist in your own town.

Many New Yorkers have never been to the top of the Empire State Building, or ridden the Staten Island Ferry. Many San Franciscans have never toured Muir Woods or the wine country.

Don't take interesting things for granted or skip visiting them just because they're in your own backyard. Ask your convention center or visitors' bureau for a list of the top sights, maps, and travel directions. There may even be some discounts and freebies in the package they send you!

731 Clear clutter quickly.

Innocent little pieces of paper can gang up on you and drive you nuts—especially when they pile up everywhere and you are trying to locate one specific item, like a bill, a prescription, someone's business card, or a child's report card.

Trying to locate that one piece of paper wastes your time, and that creates major stress. You also feel as stupid as all get-out, which is very depressing.

Here are a few ways to eliminate clutter…

• **Sort your mail at the wastebasket.** Toss anything that isn't important. If you live in a building with a mailroom, don't even carry junk mail into your home. Just throw it away immediately.

• **Put all your bills into a brightly colored folder** so that you can find them quickly when you have to pay them. Put anything that requires your immediate attention into the same or another brightly colored folder.

• **Put almost everything else into one single box or folder and deal with it every week.** Never let it overflow; that's how you got into trouble in the first place.

• **Use refrigerator magnets** for appointment slips, prescriptions, and dry-cleaning tickets.

732 Simplify your life.

This concept is broader and more profound than merely lightening your "to-do" list (Tip 711).

Think about what is really important to your life, versus what you can get along without. The excesses of Hollywood celebrities and Wall Street tycoons assault us every day through the media. But even without the collection of 100 vintage cars or 1,000 designer gowns, some of us are pack rats on a smaller, more modest scale, with three or four cars and 50 pairs of shoes.

Are all your possessions really necessary, or is it time to give away or sell some of them? *Remember*: What you don't have, you don't have to store, clean, or insure.

733 Use the five-day weather forecast.

Paying attention to the five-day forecast can simplify your planning. If you have a home-based business and live in an area where the weather varies greatly, take advantage of pleasant days to run errands and meet with clients and friends. Use nasty weather for phoning prospects and clients and working on detailed projects that need long periods of concentration.

734 Go barefoot where it's safe.

Few mood-lifters beat going barefoot. Therapists would probably say that it's a psychic return to a happy, carefree childhood. Walking barefoot in your home is safest, and wiggling your toes into plush carpets and fluffy rugs is pure, sensuous delight.

If your toes and feet are normally sensitive, without neuropathy, it may also be safe to walk barefoot on your lawn or on a pristine beach. Keep on wiggling those toes and feel like a happy kid again! (And examine your toes and feet carefully afterward.)

735 Go on a scavenger hunt.

You'll need two people or two evenly matched teams for this creative game.

First, have each person or team list 10 unusual items on a piece of paper. Next, exchange lists and agree on a time for the hunt to end and a meeting place.

Now off you go on your hunt! No swiping allowed—if you need someone's property, get permission to borrow it and make sure you return it undamaged.

The winning person or team is the one who collects the most items or, if there is a tie, the most unusual choices.

736 Have an upside-down day.

Just for fun, make a weekend day an upside-down day. Eat your dinner for breakfast—you may need to adjust your diabetes medication—and your breakfast for dinner. If you usually wear casual clothes, dress up, and vice versa.

How many other things can you do to shake up your routine a little bit?

737 Enjoy the seasons.

First snowstorm of the season? Build a snowman or have a snowball fight with your kids or your partner. Or just throw snowballs at a tree or a wall to check out your pitching arm.

Spring? Visit some of the big-city flower shows or botanical gardens. Pick up some ideas for houseplants or for your garden.

Summer? Get into a hammock or a rocking chair with some sugarless lemonade or diet soda. Ree-lax!

Fall? Go to the best or nearest place to see the leaves change color. A weekend trip with a night at a country inn would be lovely, but a drive or walk through your neighborhood can also fill your spirit with beauty.

738 Try an unusual weekend activity.

As they used to say on *Monty Python's Flying Circus*, "And now for something completely different"…

Shake up your weekend routine by trying something that's unusual for you. Do you like to visit museums or see movies? Go to a ball game instead or organize a potluck dinner with some friends. Plan your next vacation—real or imagined. Wander through an antiques show or hit the yard sales. Check the weekend edition of your newspaper for more ideas.

739 Visit a comedy club.

Comedy Central offers lots of laughs, but visiting a comedy club is much better. There is much more spontaneity, outrageousness, and topicality—and far less censorship. And there's always the chance that you'll see a major new talent at the beginning of his/her career.

740 Reality check I: Ten things you like about yourself.

When we're depressed—and people with diabetes frequently are—we focus on the negatives, not the positives. We see the glass as half-empty, not half-full.

So here's a reality check to put things in perspective. Sit down and make a list of 10 things that you like about yourself. They can focus on your appearance, your achievements, or anything else. But you *must* come up with 10. (If you need inspiration and help, ask your family and friends.)

741 Reality check II: Ten things you want to change.

Now it's time to focus on the future. Think of what you'd like to change. Maybe it's as simple as a hairstyle or color, or as complex as a career change.

Again, sit down and list the 10 things you want to change.

Remember: You can *always* make changes in your life.

742 Reality check III: If you had only one year to live.

And now here's the most intimate and challenging exercise. What would you do if you had only one year to live? How would your priorities change? What would become the most important things to do? What would you dump?

Of course, you have much more time. But separating the truly important from the trivial is necessary to get joy out of life.

Remember the old Latin motto: Carpe diem (Seize the day).

743 Make a sexy phone call.

OK, you've been serious and soul-searching long enough. Now it's time to inject some fun into your day. Make a sexy phone call to the person you love most. It could go like this:

"This is an official obscene phone call. Know what I'm gonna do to you tonight? First I'm gonna chew off all your buttons, kissing you in between each one. And then I'm gonna kiss you up, down, and sideways. And then…" You fill in the blanks if you're not both already giggling hysterically or getting hot and steamy.

744 Create a cartoon wall.

Collect your favorite cartoons and frame them if you're feeling crafty, then hang them on a wall. Use magnets to put them on the refrigerator or inside your front door.

I like putting cartoons into Lucite shadowbox frames because it's so easy to slide out old favorites and slide in new ones to create a constantly changing gallery of humor.

745 Consider a career change.

Very often unhappiness with your job is at the root of your depression or stress. Here are some things you can do about it:

If your own job gives you grief but the company and benefits are good, check with your company's bulletin boards or make a friend in the Human Resources Department and see if there are other, better jobs that you might qualify for. Network with friends at other companies; maybe they're hiring. Start reading the weekend help-wanted ads or look on the Internet for job postings. Polish up your resume.

Or, given the trends in outsourcing, maybe this is the time to go into business for yourself! (That's what I did 44 years ago.)

746 Indulge in music's "Valium" effect.

Classical music has been shown to work as well as Valium. In a study conducted at Baltimore's St. Agnes Hospital by cardiologist Raymond Bahr, MD, listening to 30 minutes of classical music had the same tranquilizing effect as 10 mg of Valium. Drift and soothe yourself with Pachelbel's *Canon*, Ravel's *Bolero*, or chamber music by Bach, Haydn, Mozart, or Beethoven.

747 Stop multitasking.

Do one thing at a time before moving on to the next job. Eliminating distractions and focusing on the task at hand will help you complete it more quickly and accurately. And focusing on one thing at a time will make you feel less stressed.

748 Carve out at least one hour a day for yourself.

Teach your kids to keep out when your door is closed, except in emergencies. (If they can close their doors, why can't you?)

Don't answer the phone—that's what answering machines and voice mail are for. This is *your* time, for just unwinding and recharging.

749 Temper, temper.

Here's a powerful reason to lower your stress level. Men who are generally hostile or frequently angry may have as much as a 30% greater risk of developing such irregular heart rhythms as atrial fibrillation, a risk factor for stroke, according to the noted Framingham Offspring Survey.

Hostility did not appear to increase heart disease in women, but researchers believe that stress can also impact men's and women's general and cardiovascular health by influencing them to practice unhealthy habits.

750 Mindfulness meditation reduces stress.

Like other forms of meditation, mindfulness meditation is an exercise in centering. In mindfulness meditation, you become deeply aware of the present moment, a practice that reduces stress and may boost immune-system function, according to a research review done at Johns Hopkins and reported in the January 6, 2014, issue of *JAMA Internal Medicine*.

To practice mindfulness meditation, sit quietly for 10 to 20 minutes, clearing all thoughts from your mind. Close your eyes and breathe deeply and evenly.

751 Make mine meditation.

In the February 9, 2015, issue of *Forbes* magazine, brilliant author Alice G. Walton wrote the well-researched article, "Seven Ways Meditation Can Actually Change the Brain"…

1. **Meditation helps preserve the aging brain.**
2. **Meditation reduces activity in the brain's "me center,"** which is responsible for the mind wandering, what the late science-fiction author Alfred Bester termed "grasshopper brain."
3. **Meditation's effects rival medication for depression and anxiety.**
4. **Meditation may lead to volume changes in key areas of the brain.**
5. **Just a few days of training improves concentration and attention.**
6. **Meditation reduces anxiety and social anxiety.**
7. **Meditation can help overcome smoking addiction.**

Other research has found that meditation training can be helpful in treating other forms of addiction.

752 Mindfulness meditation in a good book.

If you'd like an inspirational book to keep by your bedside, consider *The Mindfulness Solution: Everyday Practices for Everyday Problems* by Ronald D. Siegel, PsyD, of the Harvard Medical School. The book has many worksheets to guide you and help you focus and destress.

753 Maybe your stress is just eyestrain.

Your stress may be caused by simple eyestrain. If your stress disappears when you close your eyes or gaze out of the window for 30 seconds, eyestrain may be the culprit. When was the last time you had your vision and your eyeglasses checked? (People with diabetes should see an ophthalmologist at least every six months and an optometrist at least once a year.) Your eyeglass frames may need a little tightening or adjustment so that your eyes are looking through exactly the right area of the lenses.

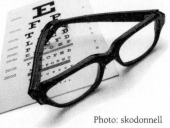

Quick fix: Soak cotton balls in undiluted witch hazel and press the compresses on your eyelids for five to 10 minutes. Even better, keep the bottle of witch hazel in your refrigerator between uses so that its cold soothes your eyes even more. (For more on diabetes and your eyes, see chapter 9.)

Photo: skodonnell

754 Color your hair.

Gray hair can be very depressing. It makes us realize that we are getting older and, visually, gray hair can wash the color out of your face.

Temporary hair colors that last through three or four shampoos are available for men as well as for women. Try one and, if you like the results and start receiving compliments from your friends, family, and especially strangers, try a permanent hair color. Life is too short to have gray hair!

755 Color your environment.

Colors awake strong emotional responses. Savvy people use them as antidepressants. You can transform the boring blandness of a white or beige room or apartment without even painting it. Create happier moods with inexpensive accessories.

A century of research into the psychology of color shows that colors have the power to evoke moods…

Blue—the most soothing, peaceful, and nurturing color. (Remember the blue of the Madonna's robe.)

Green—serene, suggestive of gardens, forests, the natural world.

Red and orange—warmth, excitement, drama.
Yellow—sunlight and optimism.

Add splashes of color to your rooms easily and quickly by hanging stained-glass suncatchers in your windows, collecting cheerful coffee mugs, choosing new towels, throws, blankets, and decorative pillows, and even——for maximum variety at minimum cost——stocking up on coordinating paper plates and napkins.

Perk up your workspace with a funny cursor and a beautiful screen saver.

756 Update Ko-Ko's list.

First a little background: In Gilbert and Sullivan's *Mikado*, Ko-Ko, the Lord High Executioner, rattles off a delightful patter song, cataloging all the types of people who irritate him, concluding each verse with "They'll none of them be missed."

The original song dates back to the 1850s, but its concept is even more timely today, and invites us to destress ourselves by updating Ko-Ko's list with our own pet peeves.

For inspiration, here is master parodist Keith Peterson's witty update…

"There's the movie palace patron with the intermittent cough;
The pest who owns a PDA and never turns it off;
The diner who is less than prompt at reaching for the check;
The broker who promotes a stock because it ends in '-tech';
And women in department stores who fill your lungs with mist—
I rather doubt the mist is likely to be missed!"

Now you try it—you'll feel a lot better!

757 Water works I: Plug it in.

Fountains possess a hypnotic quality that soothes us and lifts our spirits. Fountains have such a positive effect on us because the circulating water raises the levels of negative ions (the air's electrically charged particles) that make our spirits soar. You can find a small fountain with a compact circulating pump for your home or garden for less than $100.

758 Water works II: Crystal clear.

Water in glass containers concentrates light and energy, according to the Hindu design philosophy *vastu*. For optimal effect, arrange clear vases filled with water in powerful groups of three to represent the life-force triad: wind, water, and fire.

759 Handle curveballs with style and grace.

Life is full of potholes and curveballs. The key to your overcoming them is being flexible, rather than rigid. We all had grandmothers who dealt successfully with unexpected guests or tiny food budgets by adding more water and spices to the "always magically full" soup pot. Or friends who perfected the art of the five-minute straighten-up by piling everything behind the shower curtain.

You can always find solutions if you innovate!

760 Depression is underdiagnosed in men.

Millions of American men suffer from undiagnosed depression. Although more than six million men are estimated to have a depressive disorder, according to American Psychological Association 2015 statistics, many health professionals believe that many of these men—if not most of them—may never be treated for it. Psychological surveys continue to show that men who are depressed try to hide it with overwork; others expose themselves to harm via risky behavior. Untreated depression can result in personal, family and financial problems, even suicide. According to the National Institue of Mental Health (NIMH), four times as many men as women die by suicide in the United States. Yet eight out of 10 cases of depression respond to treatment.

Men, this may be a wake-up call to do some serious soul-searching. If you've been feeling unhappy or anxious for more than two weeks, tell your doctor that you think you may be depressed, and ask for help.

761 Practice cognitive restructuring.

We often tend to "awfulize" situations. Little things get magnified all out of proportion. Your commuter train is late two days in a row, and you automatically jump to destructive thoughts that your boss is ready to fire you.

When negative thoughts like this become an automatic response, they can lead to hypertension, depression, and other physical and emotional ills.

Cognitive restructuring (CR) is a mental technique that lessens negative thinking. It teaches you to think in context instead of "awfulizing." To practice CR, begin by saying "Stop!" to yourself. This silent command breaks the cycle of negativity. Then take two or three deep breaths and let them out slowly.

Next, give yourself a reality check: Are you seeing this situation in the worst possible light? Are there other ways to look at it? A better, more probable perspective?

Finally, take positive action: Is there an intelligent way to deal with this problem? Then do it!

762 Stop the "fat and uglies."

Emotional eating expert Geneen Roth, author of *Feeding the Hungry Heart* and *When Food Is Love*, coined the "fat and uglies," a concept that many people with diabetes are familiar with, and which increases their feelings of worthlessness and desperation, making them want to pig out beyond belief.

According to Roth, we don't know what triggers the syndrome—only that we feel so unloved that we retreat to food, the only thing that *does* love us.

The best way to disarm the fat and uglies is to have an internal dialogue with your fault-finding self. Agree with it, and you'll destroy its poisonous power. Say to yourself, "Yeah? So what?" when your "bad self" starts ranting that you're fat and ugly. When you confront yourself, you can avoid harmful emotional eating, move on, and feel like your own, good, valuable self again.

763 Cheap pampering I: Makeup makeover.

Ladies, this one's free and lots of fun. Visit a department store—especially during seasonal promotions—and get a makeup makeover. Let one of the makeup artists apply new products and colors. Usually you're not obligated to buy anything, but you may be tempted to treat yourself to a new lipstick to coordinate with the season's hot new colors.

764 Cheap pampering II: Mini massage.

You don 't need to spend an hour or $100. Many massage studios and nail salons provide 10-minute mini massages for $10 or $15, which may be all you need to relax your neck and shoulders and make you feel marvelous. You can find massage therapists who offer these quick treats at many malls and parks, or through the American Massage Therapy Association, AMTAmassage.org.

765 Cheap pampering III: Transform your bathroom.

A bathroom that appeals to your senses can feel incredibly pampering, and you can do it very inexpensively. *Here are some ideas to get you started…*

• **Spray-paint a handful of pebbles gold, so that they resemble gold nuggets.** Arrange them in a clear glass dish on your sink counter.

• **Or take some pretty shells or some colored pebbles for an aquarium and place them in the dish.**

• **Buy several cakes of scented soap.** Some—like lavender or oatmeal and almond—are unisex.

• **Buy a few loofahs and some deep-sea sponges in different sizes and textures** for your bathing and showering pleasure.

•**A little more expensive, but definitely worth it**—a new showerhead with a variety of pulse and spray options so that you can customize every shower you take.

766 Cheap pampering IV: Dress up your bedroom.

You can make your bedroom feel very special, too, and make its inhabitants feel very pampered. *Try these ideas…*

•**Put a vase with fresh, silk, or synthetic flowers on your dresser.** Or—for a touch of drama—use four or five peacock feathers, available at many flower or craft shops.

•**Place sachets in your dresser drawers and linen closet,** or line them and your closet shelves with scented paper. Here, too, lavender is an excellent unisex choice.

•**For a little splurge, pile a collection of decorative pillows on your bed.** You can usually find them on sale at home-decor shops.

767 Have you forgotten what *you* want?

Curiously, it is both a cause and an effect of stress that you may have forgotten what you like—or would like—to do. Call it the "caregiver syndrome": We are so busy taking care of other people that we forget about ourselves.

It's time for you to focus on yourself. It may have been so long since you've done so that you need some help. *List-making time…*

•**Is there anything you used to enjoy doing and would like to do again?** Anything new you'd like to try? List three films you'd like to see, three books you'd like to read.

•**Jot down the names of three friends you'd like to see more often.**

•**Write down three places where you'd like to vacation.**

768 Teach your partner or kids to do housework.

Stop being everyone's maid. It's time your family pitched in—they live there, too, and they dirty your home, too.

Many men do dishes and laundry. Teach yours to vacuum, too. Kids can set and clear the dining room table, load up the dishwasher, and even prepare dinner if they're old enough. Everyone over the age of seven should clean the bathtub after using it.

You can probably come up with a chore list more appropriate to your own family and home. This tip should start you thinking.

769 Head for the park.

A nearby park or playground offers a great escape, ideal for making your stress disappear.

Get on the swings. Climb on the jungle gym. Have fun on the seesaw.

If you're fortunate enough to have a park with a merry-go-round, take a couple of spins.

770 Whistle away stress.

Whistling, humming, or singing can melt away stress. *Here's why this happy habit works*: The sound-frequency patterns you create by making music trigger positive changes in your alpha brain waves, which relax you.

771 Beat stress—Get organized I: Stash your kitchen tools.

Putting your most frequently used kitchen utensils in a wide-mouthed jar or crock keeps them handy. Tools like tongs, spatulas, a soup ladle, a grater, baster, melon baller, and wooden spoons are easily findable in a crock, much less so if you have to rummage for them in a kitchen drawer. In fact, you can probably identify these items just from their handles.

772 Beat stress—Get organized II: Alphabetical order saves time.

This isn't a sign of obsessive-compulsive syndrome, like that of theoretical physicist Sheldon Cooper in *The Big Bang Theory*. Alphabetizing your spices and herbs saves you search time every time you cook.

773 Beat stress—Get organized III: Double your kitchen cabinet space.

Using two-tiered turntables not only doubles your cabinet space, it also makes every item on them equally accessible. That's a big time-saver!

774 Beat stress—Get organized IV: Tote your supplies easily.

Store your cleaning supplies in a caddy under the sink to carry them easily from room to room.

775 Beat stress—Get organized V: Simplify your cleaning routine.

Jot down your cleaning routine on index cards and post them on your fridge with a magnet. Try new cleaning products or methods that are supposed to save you energy and time just once, then decide whether they're worth adopting permanently. I've just bought a battery-operated set of brushes with extension handles that will save time and energy in cleaning my kitchen and bathroom.

776 Beat stress—Get organized VI: Keep backups.

Have at least one extra set of house and car keys—two sets are even better. Have alternative ways to get to work and to get the kids to school, and have several alternative babysitters.

777 Beat stress—Get organized VII: Better address books.

Add extra pages to the front of your address book and list similar people there so you can find them quickly. For example, one page might list all your doctors, the dentist, and the pharmacy, with all their addresses and phone numbers.

On another page, list all the parents in your younger child's playgroup or nursery school, and the teacher's name and phone number. A third page might list all your older child's teachers and half a dozen classmates. On a fourth page, your boss and some coworkers, and people in your car pool. On a fifth page, your mortgage holder, insurance agent, electrician, plumber, painter, handyman, and mechanic. If you have a smartphone, add descriptive information to each entry—"plumber" or "painter" or "Eva's mother"—in the title field to make finding people easier. You can also store addresses in your email program, but I find it easier to simply open a book and flip a page or two then turn on the computer.

778 Beat stress—Get organized VIII: Duplicate important documents.

Birth certificates, marriage certificates, car titles, real estate deeds, passports, and insurance policies should be protected in a safe-deposit box. Keep copies of these documents in a large plastic folder with a waterproof closure. In an emergency, just grab it and go.

779 Beat stress—Get organized IX: Nightstand necessities.

Keep these items on your nightstand within easy reach: Telephone, flashlight, pens or pencils, and a pad. You may also want to add an index card with the emergency numbers of people who are very important to you.

780 Beat stress—Get organized X: When you change the clocks, do these.

Changing your clocks back and forth to Daylight Saving Time and Standard Time is a good time to do these important little chores: Change the batteries in your smoke detector and throw out expired medicine and sunscreen.

781   Beat stress—Get organized XI: Clear your desk.

If you don't need it today, put it in your desk drawer. Keep it off your desk—you'll concentrate better.

However, if those papers and files overflow that desk drawer, it's a wake-up call that you need to do some major organizing and purging.

782   Banish toxic people from your life.

Toxic people depress us. They make us unhappy. Their negative energy poisons everyone and everything around them. If someone or something is 95% wonderful, toxic people will focus on and criticize the other 5%.

There's a simple solution: Recognize that only a miracle (or therapy?) will change these toxic people, so banish them from your life. You'll be so much happier!

783   Learn to say no.

Some people are such givers that they become stressed. They are overscheduled and overburdened.

If you are one of these saintly people, learn to say no. It's an act of self-affirmation and empowerment.

If you're not used to saying no: Learn to say "I'm sorry, but I can't." Period. No explanation. If someone presses you to explain, just repeat, "I'm sorry, but I can't."

Eventually your questioner will back off.

End of your stress.

784   Have no regrets.

Life is really too short to have regrets. As the eternally beautiful Sophia Loren is reported to have said, "I have no regrets. Regret only makes wrinkles."

785   Play the inventor.

Let your imagination run wild. What kind of product or gizmo is missing from your life? Can you make it from scratch or cobble it together from things you already have? Think about it, sketch it, and maybe even make it!

786   Make your appearance a positive.

When you feel better, you think and look better, which makes you feel better, and so on. If you feel terrible—for emotional, physical, spiritual, or any other "reasons"—clean up and dress up. Putting yourself into a downward spiral at any point will have a domino effect. If you're irritated or disgusted with yourself over food or exercise promises not kept, pulling your visible self into shape gives you more strength and motivation to begin the next step of getting to where you (or your doctors) want you to be.

787 Put your belief to work for you.

Countless studies have shown that optimism can extend your lifespan. Optimists tend to outlive pessimists, and people with religious beliefs tend to live longer than atheists. A positive outlook can make enormous differences, and using that inner strength can make controlling blood-glucose levels much easier. If you ever gave up a beloved food for Lent or stopped eating bread during Passover, then you know how much easier small self-denials can be when they're made for a Greater Cause.

788 Support networks make all the difference.

How many people love you? How many do you love? How many do you kiss and hug, and have contact with every week? Research studies show that people with strong networks of intimate social contacts are healthier, happier, and stronger, longer. If social situations are difficult for you, consider joining a club for one of your interests. Being in a room full of other bridge or chess players, or slot-car enthusiasts, or quilters, or amateur chefs, gives you many automatic conversational openings. And those contacts can boost your immune system as much as they lift your spirits.

789 When you can't do anything else, relax.

A positive attitude is more than optimism and a smile—it's sometimes the only thing you can do to make a situation better. Studies show that emotional resilience is one of the most important qualities you can bring to your health and your quality of life. So after you've done all you can, if there's nothing else you can do, relax and see where the flow takes you. Stressing yourself with no benefit will only make your situation worse, and who needs that?

790 Limit the damage by adjusting your lifestyle.

You are in control—not of everything, not of every detail. But you are in control of the *limits* of your diabetes, and that's a mantra well worth repeating. What you eat, how much you exercise, whether or not you smoke, whether you drink to excess—these behaviors accelerate or delay many complications of diabetes. In the moments when you feel restricted or resentful, remember: In large part, as much as you are willing to accept responsibility, *you* are in control.

791 Promise someone to be smart and healthy.

Tell the truth: Don't you keep promises to other people better than you keep promises to yourself? Most people do, so use it to your advantage. Promise someone special that you will develop new health habits. Be specific. For many people with diabetes, keeping that promise is easier because it has another person attached to it.

792 Get touched by an angel.

The lovely overseeing angel on the former TV series *Touched by an Angel* wants to help other people with diabetes. Actress and ordained minister Della Reese, was diagnosed with type 2 diabetes many years ago. In the summer of 2016, after celebrating her 85th birthday, she finally took control of her disease: "With diet, exercise, and medication, I took control of my diabetes. I lost 20 pounds and lowered my blood sugar from between 275 and 300 to between 67 and 110." For her inspiring story, visit DiabetesDigest.com/della-reese-staying-strong-diabetes

793 Sleep with your dog for comfort and stress reduction.

In an August 3, 2016, article in *Today* magazine, writer Meghan Holohan cited research published in a December 2015 issue of London's *Daily Mail*, finding that sleeping with your dog can help people with anxiety. They get better, more restful sleep because dogs are warm and comforting. Think of your dog as a warm, living teddy bear!

Note: I have slept with my dogs for the past 30 years. I'll vouch for their warmth, comfort, and stress reduction! But make sure your bed is big enough. Dogs can be bed hogs, too!

794 Clean windows lift your mood.

Few household things are more cheering than a clean window with the sun shining through it, especially in the winter. If cleaning them is a problem for you and you can't afford to have them done, just clean the *lower half of one window*, so that the most important part will let the sun shine in. It's a guaranteed depression-lifter!

795 Dried flowers make a beautiful permanent bouquet.

If fresh flowers aren't convenient or available, dried or fabric flowers make a pretty, permanent display, and the petals don't drop for you to have to vacuum up. Baby's breath in a colored glass vase is especially attractive.

796 Start conversations with neighbors—they may become friends.

In this era of social anxiety, which alone can cause depression and stress, starting conversations with your neighbors can do a lot to reverse this trend. It can be as simple as saying, "Hi, it's good to see you. What's happening?"

In the words of Humphrey Bogart's character Rick Blaine in *Casablanca*, "This can be the beginning of a beautiful friendship."

797 Make a rainbow to lift your spirits.

A prism from an old chandelier or from a scientific-supply store, or a crystal from a crafts shop—use any or all of them to create rainbows in the sun. They will lift your spirits!

798 "Retail therapy" can be a mood-lifter.

It's called "retail therapy" because shopping is therapeutic. Recent studies show that half of all Americans admit to following the mantra, "When the going gets tough, the tough go shopping."

Some therapeutic benefits of shopping…

•**Shopping for inspiration**—getting ideas for home and work.

•**Shopping for relaxation and escape,** while your unconscious mind works out problems.

Note: If you're a compulsive *buyer*, ignore this tip. Running up debt will only add to your stress and depression.

Undeniably, the best antidepressant and de-stresser is a "loving" relationship. To keep your love growing and glowing, try these easy ways to get romantic. I hope they inspire you to create your own rituals!

799 Get romantic I: Stargaze.

On a clear summer evening, spread out a blanket and sit under the stars. Look up at the heavens and share your dreams for the future.

800 Get romantic II: Break a sweat together.

Sweating is sexy! The aroma of your love can be a real turn-on. Go hiking or running together, or do some heavy cleaning together.

801 Get romantic III: Celebrate special anniversaries *now*.

You may or may not reach your golden anniversary, so celebrate it now—just the two of you—with a special trip, or something you've always wanted to do.

Or celebrate the anniversary of the day you met, your first date, or any occasion that's meaningful to you.

802 Get romantic IV: Read love poetry to each other.

Great poetry is very romantic, and there are thousands of beautiful, sensual poems to choose from.

My personal favorites for a romantic evening: Chilean poet Pablo Neruda's *100 Love Sonnets* (*Cien sonetos de amor*), in a bilingual edition…Shakespeare's sonnets (154 to sample!)…and poetry by e.e. cummings, Edna St. Vincent Millay, Robert Graves, Edward FitzGerald's many translations of *The Rubaiyat of Omar Khayyam*, and the poems of Gaius Valerius Catullus.

Take turns reading to each other and enjoy the sound of your beloved's voice!

803 Get romantic V: Say it's your second honeymoon.

If you're going on vacation, you can often get VIP treatment from hotels, tours, and cruise lines if you tell them it's your honeymoon. Champagne, gift baskets, and a free spa visit have all been reported by happy couples.

804 Get romantic VI: Start a collection together.

It doesn't have to be expensive or *Antiques Roadshow* or *Incurable Collector* quality. What counts is that you're doing something pleasurable together and learning together.

Start by making the rounds of yard sales and thrift shops to see if anything appeals to you—especially objects that you'd like to collect in quantity. There are lots of interesting, attractive items you can buy in the $25 to $100 range. They even may possess long-term investment potential.

805 Get romantic VII: Feast on an aphrodisiac dinner.

I won't discuss the nutritional value of my suggestions here, although they definitely exist. What's important is their delicious decadence and their deserved centuries-old reputations as aphrodisiacs. *Also, as you don't want to spend hours in the kitchen, you can put this entire meal together in less than half an hour…*

Brut (very dry) champagne—or domestic sparkling wine is fine.

Caviar—salmon roe is tasty and inexpensive.

Lobster or crabmeat salad—make this the day before with canned crabmeat if you're on a budget.

Fresh strawberries—even if they're out of season. Dipping them in bittersweet chocolate before you feed them to each other will make them even more decadent!

806 Get romantic VIII: Spend a day in bed with your love.

The best for last! Lock the door and turn off the phone. 'Nuff said!

CHAPTER 7

Tips for Children with Diabetes and Their Parents

Pediatric diabetes comes in all sizes and ages, from the baby girl written about in Dr. Tamler's thoughtful Foreword on up to adolescents verging on adulthood. Therefore, some of these tips will be useful to some age groups, some to all age groups, and some even to diabetic adults.

807 Know the link between childhood obesity and pediatric diabetes.

Pediatric diabetes not only hits early, but is often more severe, owing to childhood obesity. "Children are coming in with diabetes in their teens," says Jane Kim, MD, a pediatric endocrinologist at the University of California-San Diego School of Medicine. "Their parents might have been diagnosed in their 30s or 40s, and their grandparents in their 50s and 60s."

Type 2 diabetes in children often has such severe complications as kidney disease, eye disease, and nerve damage.

Prevent your children from obesity to prevent or forestall type 2 diabetes, even though it's extra work for all of you. It will definitely pay off!

808 Monitor blood glucose frequently.

A Children with Diabetes* poll from November 2013 reported that 89% of patients checked their blood glucose more than six times a day, and 40% checked it at least 10 times a day. If you have rapidly growing toddlers or children, this is the ounce of prevention to avoid that future pound of care.

809 Practice nighttime blood-glucose testing.

In a Children with Diabetes poll from March 2013, 34% of readers reported checking nighttime blood-glucose levels every night, while 48% reported checking at least once a week. Nighttime checking makes good sense, espe-

*Children with Diabetes is a not-for-profit online community for kids, families, and adults with diabetes.

205

cially for young children whose brains are developing rapidly. Furthermore, growing evidence points to more nocturnal hypoglycemia than previously thought, and to a greater number of problems associated with nocturnal hypoglycemia like falls and seizures.

810 Ouch!!!

According to the Children with Diabetes Foundation, if your five-year-old is diagnosed with type 1 diabetes, he or she will have endured *at least 18,980 finger sticks* to test blood glucose by the age of 18.

    Two suggestions: Rotate the sticking sites on all eight fingers—but *do not use your child's thumbs!*

    And give your diabetic child some extra TLC.

811 Get some support.

Nobody will understand your situation and frustrations like another parent with a diabetic child—and you may not need to reinvent any wheels someone else has already discovered. Log on to ChildrenWithDiabetes.com for an online community for kids, families, and adults with diabetes. News of breakthroughs, upcoming conferences, nutrition, summer camps, basics, and warning signs—this is a fine website to start with or return to. For adult resources check Diabetes.org.

812 Financial help is available in emergencies.

Families struggling to pay for diabetes supplies have places to turn for assistance. For example, children with type 1 diabetes who are in emergency situations—like the loss of health insurance, loss of a parent's job, or a local disaster—can get supplies. This program is part of the American Board for Child Diabetics. For more information, log on to ChildrenWithDiabetes.com and go to Scholarships and Financial Aid.

813 Your child's diabetes requires cooperation from caregivers.

If your child is in day care or school, make sure that your child's teacher knows you need their help with reinforcing healthy eating habits away from home. Schools with cafeterias publish their daily menus ahead of time; offer healthy snacks to share with the class on days when it's your child's turn to bring treats. And send him off armed with a healthy lunch and snack on days when the school's foods aren't appropriate for his diet.

814 Because you're the parent—that's why.

Frustrating and inconvenient as it can be sometimes, you're a grown-up, and it's important to help your child manage his/her diabetes successfully. Teaching your child how to eat properly now will set patterns that will help him manage his diabetes for the rest of his life.

The healthy eating plan you adopt for your diabetic child can be good for your entire family to follow. Your commitment to your child's present and future well-being must be full-blown and full-time. Even more than telling him what's right and counting his exchanges and helping to monitor his blood-glucose levels, you need to display behavior worthy of copying. Eat your six-plus servings of fresh fruits and vegetables every day. Skip the gravy on your entree, so he learns that it's tasty without the "goo." And if you *must* have a candy bar, indulge when your child is in school or somewhere else that you're not. He'll learn much more from what he sees you *do* than from what he hears you say.

815 More water, please.

Teach your child to drink water as the beverage of choice. Good hydration helps the body control blood-glucose levels, and water also helps limit carbohydrate intake from other beverages. Drinking eight ounces of orange juice is the carbohydrate equivalent of eating two oranges; choosing eight ounces of water instead will do your child twice as much good, with no calories or carbohydrates.

816 What a friend we have in fiber.

There are many reasons why increasing your child's fiber intake will benefit his/her body. Your grandma told you about roughage; enough said there! But in addition to moving waste through the intestines more quickly, high-fiber foods are more satisfying because they are so filling. They are digested more slowly, and they keep blood-glucose levels more consistent for longer.

Give your child more fiber without his even noticing. Try substituting high-fiber foods like whole-grain bread or cereal, beans, and popcorn for white breads, sugary cereals, and potato chips.

817 Make TV a dirty word.

Studies show that the more time kids spend watching television, the more likely they are to be overweight—and to eat poorly. These are the key causes of the pandemic of type 2 diabetes in children and adolescents.

Make TV a treat, blocking out time only for certain programs or special occasions, the one or two shows that your child really wants to see.

In addition to limiting sedentary viewing time, there's an added bonus: Your child learns to set priorities and limits by ranking chosen favorites over "whatever's on at 7:00."

818 Ban eating in front of the TV.

Make this a family rule, and keep it: No eating anywhere, except in the kitchen or dining room. Snacks in front of the tube are doubly deadly. Not only are you and your kids zoned out and sedentary, you're also consuming calories that are almost certainly carbs and fats. And people tend to eat more when they're watching TV than when sitting at a table. (Admit it: Nobody eats celery sticks in front of the boob tube.) And unless you have a dog to police the area for you, those Cheetos hidden in the sofa cushions are the perfect bug bait!

819 Sneak some vegetables into your kids.

Even if they "hate vegetables," you can disguise them and slip them into other dishes, and they won't even realize they're eating healthier.

Add cut-up extra vegetables to chili or stir-fry dishes. Grate root vegetables like carrots and turnips and add them to stews. (Don't sneer until you've tried it—you really won't taste them!)

And when you eat these added veggies, *your* skin will start glowing, too!

820 Do this sneaky substitution.

Many kids dislike cauliflower, but they love rice. OK, then, fool them for their own good. Grating raw cauliflower on a cheese grater or pulsing in a food processor will make it into little rice-shaped nuggets that you can then cook for three minutes or so in a frying pan with a little olive oil. When the cauliflower is soft, fluff it with a fork. Serve it up as is, or with a little tomato or cheese sauce. Your kids will get vitamins and fiber in a tasty side dish that looks like rice—without all the carbs.

821 Pick fruit first.

As soon as diabetic toddlers develop teeth, offer them chunks of fresh fruit. They will enjoy manipulating this new finger food, and fresh fruit has more nutrients and fiber than juice, and won't make their blood glucose rise as rapidly because it is digested more slowly.

Save the fruit juice for their hypoglycemic episodes.

822 Your child's medication will change.

As kids grow, they gain weight. Their diets change, and so may their activity level.

Diabetic kids are no different. Any one of these changes will alter their insulin and other drug needs.

Phone your child's pediatrician or endocrinologist if your child is starting a growth spurt, beginning school, or if you simply find that your child's formerly predictable blood-glucose readings are yo-yoing.

823 Let all the teachers know your child's needs.

Diabetes requires a great deal of monitoring and self-care. Diabetic schoolchildren often depend on teachers and staff to provide the encouragement and support they need to take care of themselves. Be sure your child's teachers—*all* of them, not just homeroom—know that he needs extra bathroom breaks, and specific times to check blood-glucose levels and have a snack.

Don't let an overworked teacher or snippy administrator tell you she can't take on any additional obligations—schools have a legal responsibility to accommodate the special needs of children with diabetes.

824 Diabetes at school can mean more than snacks and monitoring.

Diabetic children may need special understanding. Their concentration can wander, and occasional behavior difficulties can arise out of rapid changes in blood-glucose levels. Make sure that your child's teachers or day-care providers are educated about your child's potential emotional as well as physical needs—your child's misbehavior may not come from the same impetus as other children's, and needs to be addressed differently. Make sure your child receives fair and appropriate treatment from his teachers and school.

825 Get information or help for your child's school.

"Discrimination" sounds like an odd term for schoolchildren with diabetes, but many of today's overcrowded and overburdened school systems don't look forward to "special-needs students." You may need to educate yourself about your child's legal rights, and enlighten the school's personnel about their responsibilities toward him. Children with diabetes have to be medically safe at school and day care, while having the same access to educational opportunities as other children. The American Diabetes Association (Diabetes.org) and the Juvenile Diabetes Research Foundation (JDRF.org) provide educational materials for both parents and school personnel to understand how to meet the medical and academic needs of students with diabetes. (See Tips 870–874 for details.)

826 Yesterday's levels are history—check again and again.

Children's blood-glucose levels need to be checked often because their levels of play and food intake change so frequently. Until you establish a regular schedule, you'll know best how often your individual child needs to be checked by watching her mood and behavior, energy output at play (active versus sedentary), or even by noticing the fruity smell of her breath or urine.

Teenagers' body chemistry is in almost-constant flux, so expect that puberty may cause even more variation in blood-glucose readings, calling for more frequent testing—at least every four hours.

827 **Planning a "family sweet" twice a week takes the sting out.**

Few things spark cravings more strongly than the feelings of restriction or denial. Help your child moderate her consumption of sweets by planning special desserts once or twice a week, and making a family occasion out of sharing them. (You can decide whether a low-carb or no-sugar-added dessert is all right for other nights of the week.) By also encouraging half-sized portions, your child can feel included in a collective celebration and still indulge a little. And knowing that she's "saving up" for when the entire family can share the occasion can help with self-control at other times during the week.

828 **What your child *doesn't* eat also matters.**

Remember to give yourself points for what your child *didn't* eat today. While what he *did* consume is what shows up on the glucose meter, every sweet or fatty food would have caused more trouble in his arteries or capillaries in another decade. Controlling your child's food intake can be an overwhelming job—especially if your child isn't cooperating much yet—and parents may need to praise themselves for how good a job they do, especially on a day when they feel the job could have been done better.

829 **Develop your own Rescue Strategy.**

Keeping a level head is as important—and sometimes even more important—than keeping level blood-sugar numbers. Some parents report that the enormity of monitoring a child's blood glucose 24/7 hits them hard periodically.

Just as you have insulin or orange juice ready in case your child has a crisis, be sure you have your own "emergency fix" at hand in case you feel the blues coming on. A parents' support group, someone who can give you half a day off, even a half-hour off for a massage or a walk can make an enormous difference in your equilibrium. Keeping yourself on an even keel is the best thing you can do for your child. Just like the flight attendants' instructions, put on your own oxygen mask first so you can be in a position to help your child.

830 Even little changes can make enormous differences.

Small changes in growing children can reap enormous long-term health benefits. In preadolescent children, every inch they have yet to grow will be accompanied by pounds they have yet to gain. If your child can gain a little less weight as he approaches his final height, that growth will actually be realized as a weight loss—achieved more easily than conventional *weight loss* will ever be again, as an adult.

831 Puberty: A tough time for type 2.

A steady relationship with a good pediatrician is vital as your child grows up. Puberty in prediabetic children can bring on more body changes than the ones you'd expect. Your overweight, sedentary child's body is more insulin-resistant during puberty, and her growth spurts and weight gain during that time strain the body to produce more insulin than it can manufacture. Type 2 (insulin-resistant) diabetes can be the result, which gives your child that much more to cope with during an already-stressful part of life.

832 Diet, exercise, and insulin are the only tools for type 2 kids.

Children who develop type 2 diabetes have three easily accessed tools to treat it: Diet, exercise, and insulin.

Unfortunately, they are the only tools. The oral medications adults can use to assist insulin uptake are not approved by the FDA for use in children.

The most recent surveys indicate that one in three American children is seriously overweight—more than half in some ethnic groups like Hispanics and Native Americans. As a result, children are increasingly developing what was once labeled "adult-onset" diabetes, and may need to take insulin injections for a while, until their blood-glucose levels are stabilized. The FDA is currently studying oral drugs for use in children but, as of mid-2017, the drugs have not yet been approved.

833 Learn the new dirty words: "Escalator" and "Elevator."

Trade no-effort conveyances for stairs whenever possible. Escalators and elevators burn no calories and contribute nothing to cardiovascular health. Young children can play counting games, take stairs two at a time, or one step for each syllable of a song; older children can be "dared" or "raced" up steps. As five flights is daunting for anyone, promise your child that you'll climb one flight and then take escalators or elevators the rest of the way. Eventually, try alternating climbing one flight and riding one floor until you've reached your destination.

Don't forget to praise *any* new effort. Even eight or 10 steps in a flight of stairs really is a big accomplishment for a heavy child.

834 The real "bargain" is paying for only what you need.

The suggestion to "supersize" is everywhere, and twice as many french fries for just 99 cents more sounds like a real bargain—especially to a youngster who's good at math. The problem is that neither you nor your child need so many, and there's an extra 300 calories or more in that larger portion. If some inner sense of thrift urges either of you to buy the bigger one because it costs less, think again. Redefine "bargain" as "getting exactly what I want and need for my money." If paying a little for a lot more still excites you, then supersize your sugar-free drink and ask for a courtesy cup. Share it with your child, and both of you can skip the fries!

835 You are what you drink.

Many overweight children are telling the truth when they protest, "But I don't eat that much!" Unfortunately, kids today think nothing of downing 32-ounce "Big Gulp" drinks—the equivalent of four servings. Merchandisers have accustomed us to giant helpings, which now look normal and make six- and eight-ounce drinks look midget-sized. Teens who down two 32-ounce drinks a day have consumed one-half gallon of liquid, and even if it's fruit juice—don't let it be soda pop!—that's still an enormous load of calories and sugar. If you're determined to fork over money for a drink for your child, try low-fat milk or bottled water.

836 Indulge in half-nude burgers.

The hardest part of dietary restrictions for kids can be the sense of not being included—not being able to go to the same places and eat what their friends eat. So if a fast-food place is where the gang is going, diabetic teens can have their hamburgers along with everyone else. Just have them ask for no "special sauce"—they can use mustard or a tiny smear of ketchup and jettison half the bun. Using it like a holder, or like peeling a banana, they can tear away the bread as they eat the meat. If any jerky companion questions the practice, just have your child say, "It's soggy, it's too gross to eat!" Nobody argues with "gross!"

Better yet, have your kid toss *both* halves of the bun!

837 Know the risks of childhood type 2 diabetes.

Complications of type 2 diabetes can occur at any time, but it's worth remembering that some complications might not crop up until 20 or 30 years later. When an adult develops type 2 diabetes in her 40s, that means trouble in her late 60s and 70s. But when a 15-year-old has high blood-glucose levels, high cholesterol, and high triglycerides, that means a 35-year-old will be facing life-or-death problems related to diabetes.

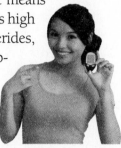

If you can see the sense of saving now for your child's college education, then it surely makes sense to take steps now to fend off her possible cardiovascular and stroke problems just 10 years after college.

Photo: RyanKing999

838 It's not "just a cold" anymore.

Diabetic children's colds and other viruses are different from other children's even if it's the same germ. Over-the-counter medicines often contain some form of sugar, and they affect blood-glucose levels and blood pressure differently in children with diabetes. Consequently, parents of diabetic children shouldn't try to self-medicate when their kids are sick. It's not trivial—call your pediatrician, and monitor blood glucose often.

839 Every kind of sick isn't the same.

It's crucial to monitor your child's blood-glucose levels if she's not well, and be prepared for both too-high and too-low readings. The stress of infection, like flu, could shoot up your child's sugar numbers. But if she's vomiting, or has a poor appetite and doesn't want to eat, then her numbers could be very low. If your child is nauseous and has hypoglycemia, flat *nondiet* cola won't upset her stomach and will raise her blood sugar.

Children with type 1 diabetes may need insulin so they don't develop ketones in their blood, but children with type 2 usually don't face that risk of ketoacidosis (a dangerous condition in which the body breaks down its own fat, releasing ketones into the blood), so their illness is usually not as serious. Nonetheless, monitor blood glucose frequently in either case!

840 Sick or well, type 1 children always need insulin.

Children who need insulin injections *always* need *some* insulin—even when they're sick and not eating. Without insulin, the body breaks down its own fat, causing ketoacidosis. How much insulin is determined by the results of their blood-glucose readings and your pediatrician's instructions.

841 Prevention is easier than treatment.

Type 2 diabetes used to be known as "adult-onset," but that name no longer holds true, as depicted in *Time* magazine's April 27, 2010, cover story, "Childhood Obesity and Diabetes: Two Sides of the Same Coin." More than 30 million people in the United States are affected by diabetes, and nearly half of all new cases are actually preteens and adolescents. The majority of type 2 children don't show many symptoms and may feel fine. If your child is heavy and sedentary, it may be possible for you to assess your child's possible risk level simply by observing his/her diet and activity level.

Because obese children have much more fat on and in their bodies, they have to produce a lot more insulin to maintain blood-glucose levels. Years of being overweight can actually exhaust the insulin-producing cells that have been working so hard for so long.

842 Dark patches can be red flags.

Overweight children who develop darkened and thickened patches on the skin around their armpits, waistline, or at the base of the neck need to be checked *immediately* for type 2 diabetes. This skin change is called *acanthosis nigricans*, and it's one of the few visible signs of diabetes. A urine test is inexpensive, painless, and very wise for children whose family history includes obesity or diabetes. (Alternatively, finger stick tests can help to detect diabetes even earlier, as you don't spill glucose into urine until blood glucose is above 200 mg/dL) So if you've scrubbed your child's "dirty neck" until it's red and it still doesn't look clean, visit your pediatrician to see whether this skin marker is a symptom of diabetes.

843 It's a head-scratcher.

If your child scratches his head a lot, it might not be deep thinking. The scalp perspires, like the skin on the rest of the body, and diabetics' perspiration can contain high sugar levels, just like their blood. That means your child's playing outside in the heat and sunshine can unwittingly create a perfect medium for an itchy yeast infection of the scalp. Encourage showers or baths with shampoo after outdoor recreation.

844 Are you sure it's "just" bed-wetting?

If your child suddenly begins wetting the bed after previously being toilet-trained and staying dry at night, check for diabetes. While stresses from school or home or other sources can affect this behavior, bed-wetting in a child who didn't have that behavior before can be a symptom of diabetes—especially if your child needs to urinate frequently during the day.

845 One little change, over and over, equals a big difference.

Make sure your child receives praise and encouragement for even small behavior changes because they can add up fast. Not drinking one can of soda can
save 150 calories; giving up one can a day can add up to a 15-pound weight
loss in a year. Make sure he knows that every bit counts!

846 It's a bit late for genes, but not too late to set a good example.

The genes your child has inherited are what they are, but the lifestyle he's
learning can be a major factor, too. Statistically, if both parents are overweight,
obese, or have type 2 diabetes and your child is overweight, he has a 90%
chance of developing diabetes. So family examples of exercise and moderate
eating habits help more than just the one person who's exercising and eating
wisely.

847 Your child catches your attitude.

Your behaving in matter-of-fact and unmartyred ways is vital to managing
your child's diabetes. Even with an oppositional toddler, your child is learning
his attitude from watching you and your attitude.

It's also vital not to blame yourself. While you couldn't have prevented
your child's condition, you can prevent or delay future complications by exercising care and lifestyle choices. And if your diabetic child has brothers or
sisters, adopting healthy eating and exercise for all of them is the best present
you can give yourself and your family.

848 Diabetes takes work and care, but it's not a stopper.

Children with diabetes can do anything any other child can do—except gorge
on carbohydrates. Sports, hiking, bike riding, dancing—as long as your child
is testing her blood glucose and taking her medication, diabetes doesn't have
to stop her from any activity she did before she was diagnosed. Of course,
watchfulness and monitoring are key, but careful eating and preparation before exertion can let diabetic children be kids.

849 Be sure your child's friends know diabetes isn't contagious.

Children are naturally curious, and your child's need for testing and injections
will naturally raise peers' questions. Head off those questions by educating
your child's friends and classmates. Most often, other children's concerns are
whether they can "catch diabetes" from your child. Once information removes
that worry, your child may discover that his peers are actually impressed. Depending on their ages, the rituals—doing blood tests and taking injections or

using an insulin pump—or even the self-discipline involved in self-care may elevate your child in his friends' estimation.

It shouldn't be necessary, but in this imperfect world, you may have to educate your child's friends' parents, too, that diabetes is not contagious.

850 Rehearse your reactions to bad behavior so you are prepared.

Sometimes a tantrum is just a tantrum. Sometimes it's the result of out-of-whack blood sugar. As the parent, you have the astounding 24/7 job of needing to reassert control in bad situations and, even harder, to react properly to your child's episodes of misbehavior.

This can be much easier if you have rehearsed your reactions mentally during calmer moments. Decide now what you would do in (a) a private or (b) a public place; whether your child needs to eat or run off some energy… has sneaked a forbidden snack…needs insulin…or is taking advantage of the situation in inconvenient but age-appropriate ways. Having a Plan A, B, C, D, and Q already formulated can save you from a great deal of guilt from having reacted in a way that you later regret.

Punishment won't change your child's blood-glucose number and consequently won't change the offending behavior, but a hard candy won't improve his attempts to manipulate you, either.

851 Make your infant's bed a safe space.

Having your infant diagnosed with diabetes can be emotionally overwhelming, but you can take some consolation and comfort in knowing that you have more help from technology and science than any parent before you. Your specialist/pediatrician can advise you about adjusting your child's insulin program around her eating—not vice versa—and can also discuss using topical anesthetics to minimize the pain and fear of finger sticks.

Most important, *never* give blood-glucose tests or injections while your child is in her crib! For better sleep, feelings of security, and many other reasons, she needs to know that her bed is a "safe space."

852 It's always easier when you play.

A huge part of a parent's job is teaching your diabetic child self-care. Just because it's responsible, it doesn't have to be dry or boring. Play—at your child's level—can be a wonderful teaching tool. Pretend-tests and show-me demonstrations on toys can make teaching necessary tasks more fun.

In fact, several companies even make dolls and teddy bears designed to teach children about diabetes. One such toy is Rufus, the Bear with Diabetes™, developed by a woman whose son was diagnosed with type 1 diabetes when he was three years old. (Rufus has since been joined by his sister Ruby, for little girls.)

For information on Rufus, the Bear with Diabetes™ and Ruby, the Bear with Diabetes™ contact the Juvenile Diabetes Research Foundation, JDRF.org.

853 Wouldn't it be great to have just the "customary" food issues?

Many toddlers have "food issues," using not-eating as a control technique as they explore their power and development.

Your diabetic child's food issues are more immediate, with bigger stakes—but never let your child force you into letting her eat what she wants just because she knows you need her to eat *something*.

One technique many parents find helpful is offering limited choices among options they have preselected. Asking, "Do you want oatmeal?" provokes a "No!" Asking "Do you want half an orange or half an apple?" gives your child some choice, and a feeling of power over his environment. And you have also gotten some good fruit into him without a struggle or major battle.

854 Don't underestimate "making mom and dad happy."

Children seek parental approval, and it's possible to encourage their compliance without turning them into "approval junkies."

Make sure that your child receives *more* positive attention for cooperating than negative attention for rebelling. To a young child, *any* attention is welcome, regardless of whether it's positive or negative. If the volume and intensity levels go up in your home when he's not complying or following instructions, he'll learn to control your household by *not* controlling his blood-glucose results. Praise his correct behaviors and choices as specifically and as often as possible—you'll both be happier than if you yell every time something is "wrong."

855 Fewer choices mean less stress.

Take a tip from actors and directors: Planning and rehearsal can save you quarts of stomach acid! Predetermine and limit your child's choices for testing times, injection sites, and snacks, and present *your* predefined options as choices. Questions like, "Do you want to test before or after you call Grandma for five minutes?" and "Do you want to try your right middle finger or your left one this time?" can minimize the stress involved in the procedure. These options give your child some control, and no big multiple-choice questions need to be answered.

856 Popeye was right!

Children often turn up their noses at spinach, so that's where Popeye comes in. After watching a couple of Popeye cartoons, boys especially are more interested in eating raw spinach in a salad, or steamed in a tasty sauce.

857 Pack your preschooler's backpack.

Ask the parents of almost any four- or five-year-old: That sweet little munchkin is a pure energy machine, with totally erratic energy levels and exertion patterns. That makes preschoolers especially vulnerable to hypoglycemia and all its problems and dangers. Make sure your child's backpack always contains protein and carbohydrate snacks or glucose tablets in order to cover any eventuality.

Suggestions: Ask your child whether she would prefer cheese, turkey slices, or almond or peanut butter on thin-sliced rye bread or crispbread, yogurt, or fresh fruit.

858 It's a number and a consideration—don't make it "good" or "bad."

Whatever numbers come up in your child's blood-glucose test results, be careful not to assign them moral values! A number isn't "good" or "bad"—it might be "higher than we'd like," or "right on target," or "a sign that we need to be more careful."

Labeling eating or test results as "good" or "bad" sets up food and esteem issues and the foundations of eating disorders that can last a lifetime.

859 Kids benefit from tight blood-glucose control.

When older children keep their blood-glucose levels within the range that their pediatricians or endocrinologists recommend, their concentration is enhanced and their schoolwork improves.

Most doctors, however, feel that infants and toddlers benefit from a wider range of blood-glucose levels in order to prevent rapid-onset hypoglycemia and frequent trips to the emergency room. Check with your child's doctors and have them tailor the appropriate range to your child.

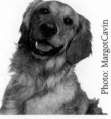
Photo: Margot Cavin

860 Your dog can be your first alarm.

Let your dog sleep in your child's bedroom. We're not copying Nana, the Saint Bernard nursemaid in *Peter Pan*, but a dog's keen sense of smell will pick up much more quickly than you can that a child with very high or very low blood sugar just smells different than usual. In fact, infants' and toddlers' wet diapers smell different to your dog, too.

When your dog wakes you in the middle of the night to take care of your diabetic child, reward it with a treat to reinforce this lifesaving behavior.

Admittedly, my evidence is anecdotal, based on stories from fellow diabetics and parents of children with diabetes. But I can tell you that my dog wakes me if my blood glucose tanks in the middle of the night. And many researchers have discovered that dogs can smell cancer, which to them apparently smells different from normal tissue.

You can learn much more about Diabetic Alert Dogs and training programs at DiabeticAlertDogsofAmerica.com.

861 Help your child win the pizza wars.

Kids love pizza, and kids with diabetes are no exception.

You don't want your child to be left out when the crowd heads for the pizzeria, but you want to protect her. The major problem is that pizza's carb-loaded crust can raise blood-glucose levels for as long as 48 hours.

If your child has an insulin pump, ask her doctor for the proper dosage of baseline and spaced boluses to balance her high blood sugars. Her doctor will also be able to calculate her dosage of rapid-acting and long-acting insulins if she uses insulin syringes or pens.

If your child is self-disciplined, urge her to eat only the pizza topping and maybe *only one bite of the crust*. Then she'll be able to have a marvelous time with her friends without wrecking her blood glucose.

862 Stay away from sneaky spaghetti sauce.

Spaghetti sauce can be sneaky! Tomato-based pasta sauce may have a lot of vitamins A and C and lycopene, a valuable antioxidant. But commercially produced brands are often loaded with sugar, high-fructose corn syrup, and sodium. Sauce from a jar can sound healthy, and it's an easy meal, but it's also dangerous for a child with diabetes.

Read the label: Even one-half cup of Prego Fresh Mushroom Italian sauce contains 11 grams of sugar and nearly half the recommended daily sodium allowance for a child. If you have the time and are feeling creative, you and your child can make your own, super-healthy spaghetti sauce in a blender or food processor, eliminating any sugar.

863 Strategize birthday parties.

Birthday parties, which are such happy occasions for nondiabetic children, can be frustrating events for diabetic children and their parents—especially if your little darling is invited to several parties every month.

The major problem is that so many carbohydrates are served within two or three hours—like pizza *and* birthday cake *and* ice cream *and* chips *and* pretzels.

Not letting your child go to parties is a major mistake. It isolates him, making him unhappy and resentful, and makes him hate his disease—all guaranteed to create anything from a temper tantrum to a problem child.

Instead, work with your child's pediatrician or endocrinologist on how to balance all those carbohydrates with additional units of fast-acting insulin—some before the party, some several hours later or even the next day.

And ask the birthday child's mother what she's going to serve so that you and your child can plan ahead.

Depending on your child's age, intelligence, and understanding, you may be able to persuade him that the best part of the birthday cake is the cake; the icing is much too sugary and can be scraped off. The chips and pretzels can be saved for another day. Offer ice cream later in the week as a family treat.

You will probably need the experience of five or six birthday parties in order to calculate the correct amount and timing of insulin for most parties, but that's a very small price to pay for your child's enjoying all those social activities.

864 Train a third adult to take care of your child.

You and your spouse or partner have already been trained how to test your child's blood glucose, how to calculate her insulin requirements, how and where to inject the insulin or use a pump, and how to recognize and treat hypoglycemia.

Unfortunately, that means that one of you is on 24/7 duty all the time.

Your love relationship needs some private time, too. And most parents of diabetic children discover that they haven't been able to get away for a romantic weekend since their child was first diagnosed—often several years ago. If you can train a third adult—a grandparent, relative, or close friend—to care for your child, you will be able to vacation by yourselves for at least a weekend at a time, and come back relaxed and refreshed.

865 Send your kid to diabetes summer camp.

Having diabetes does not exclude your child from summer camp, a core childhood experience. In fact, camps for diabetic kids started in the 1920s, just a few years after insulin became available. Now there are such camps in every state in the United States, every province in Canada, and in many developed countries. Look for diabetes camps state-by-state at Diabetes.org.

Diabetic children learn a great deal from attending these special summer camps. Most importantly, they develop independence, self-confidence, athletic abilities, and comfort and knowledge that in this society—at least—*all* the kids have diabetes.

These camps have medical staffs consisting of doctors, nurses, and dietitians. The counselor-camper ratio is high, and counselors are trained and experienced in reacting to potential blood-glucose difficulties.

There are day camps for younger children with diabetes and sleep-away camps for older ones (usually ages seven to 17). Some camps offer family programs, and many camps provide partial or full scholarships, depending on need.

When choosing a camp for your child, make sure that the medical staff checks all campers during the night to detect and correct any blood-glucose problems.

866 Walk your child to school.

Walking your child to school gives both of you some more exercise. It's also a wonderful opportunity for serious or playful one-on-one discussions.

867 Praise your child's other achievements.

Is your child gifted academically? Musically? Athletically? Has he or she earned badges in the Boy Scouts or Girl Scouts? Been elected to class office?

Emphasize *these* achievements over those related to diabetes and blood-glucose control. Concentrate on the *rest* of your child's life, not on the diabetic part, which already receives a lot of attention.

868 Question that squirming I.

If your school-age daughter squirms a lot in her chair, ask if she's "itching in private places." The sugar that spills over into diabetics' urine makes girls more susceptible to urinary tract and vaginal infections like monilia, a yeast infection. If she seems to have a recurrence of these problems, no matter how young she is, have her blood-glucose levels checked. She may need more insulin!

Boys with diabetes can have urinary tract infections, too, but they are far more common in girls.

869 Question that squirming II.

Is your child squirming in his seat, or hesitating to go to the toilet? Many books warn parents to look for intestinal parasites in children's feces. Pin-

221

worms are thin little white—sometimes wiggling—threadlike creatures in the stool. But a urinary tract infection (UTI) can be more uncomfortable or painful, and is more likely because of the high sugar content of your child's urine. If your child puts off going to the bathroom, have the doctor make sure he—or she—doesn't have a UTI.

870 Make sure the teacher and school know what's required.

The Individuals with Disabilities Education Act (IDEA) and Section 504 of the Rehabilitation Act of 1973 both protect children who have disabilities against discrimination. They are supposed to ensure that all children can take part in all school activities, and still handle their medical needs. If your child's school staff doesn't make the necessary provisions, take the attitude that they need educating, and do it gently. Indignation—even righteous indignation—will make opponents of the very people whose assistance you need.

871 Request an individualized education program…it's not "Special Ed."

Every school that receives federal funding must comply with the Individuals with Disabilities Education Act (IDEA). That means you can request an Individualized Education Program (IEP) and a Section 504 Accommodation for your child, and the school staff must meet with you about your child's special needs. Updated April 15, 2015, the School Bill of Rights for Children with Diabetes website (ChildrenWithDiabetes.com) includes a seven-point list of services. *Here it is, so you don't miss anything that could assist your child…*

1. Do blood sugar checks when and where they want.

2. Treat hypoglycemia with emergency sugar.

3. Inject insulin when necessary.

4. Eat snacks when necessary.

5. Eat lunch at an appropriate time and have enough time to finish the meal.

6. Have free and unrestricted access to water and the bathroom.

7. Participate fully in physical education (gym class) and other extracurricular activities, including field trips.

872 Where to begin when talking to opposing forces.

Most schools are clear on their responsibilities to children with diabetes, as per the Individuals with Disabilities Education Act (IDEA), which guarantees that your child can care for his diabetes while in school. Many school systems can no longer afford full-time school nurses, but they are required to allow your child time and opportunity for blood-glucose self-testing, unrestricted access to drinking water and the bathroom, snacks as needed, participation in gym classes and field trips, and the privacy and opportunity to inject insulin when necessary.

If your child's school refuses to comply, your first step should be to file a complaint with your local Board of Education. If you aren't satisfied with the Board's response, contact your state's department of education.

873 The flip side of privilege is responsibility.

Your child must be permitted to bring syringes to school if she injects insulin, but she also needs to be responsible about their disposal after use. Your notifying the school's officials—plus your child's responsible behavior regarding syringes' use and disposal—will distinguish her "needles" from any of the administration's fears about "drug paraphernalia."

Note: The needles for injecting insulin are *much* too short to inject illicit drugs.

874 Assume they're misinformed, rather than insensitive morons.

If your child's school administration isn't cooperative about the special needs of his diabetes, be as gracious as possible for as long as you can before invoking the legal system. The U.S. Department of Education Office for Civil Rights (OCR) has an official Discrimination Complaint Form.

It comes in two varieties accessible from its website: A PDF that you can print, fill out and mail back, or you can file your complaint electronically. Go to Ed.gov/about/offices/list/ocr/complaintintro.html. And be sure to make a copy for your own file!

Your child's medical condition mandates nondiscriminatory treatment—but exhaust all other possibilities before making a literal federal case of it. Be aware that filing a complaint is the first step to litigation, which could cause your child some day-to-day friction at school with administrators, teachers, or smart-mouthed peers.

875 "Fair" is about everyone getting what they need.

Children have innate fairness-sensing mechanisms, and some are not above using claims of perceived unfairness as a manipulation tool. Your child's individual snacks or extra bathroom privileges may be what's inspiring any jealousy from other students. Should she run into classmate complaints about her "extra privileges," don't burden her self-esteem further by trying to "even up the score" by pointing out the disadvantages of her condition. Instead, instruct your child to tell bullies and teases that "fair" means everybody gets what they need, and not everybody needs the same thing.

876 One page is best for instructions.

Most children's special diabetic needs during school can be listed, double-spaced, on one page. Giving your child's teacher a single sheet makes it easy to read, post, and reread in a rushed or worried moment, and copies can easily be given to the school's principal, nurse, and secretaries.

Make it as easy as possible for others to assist your child. Your goal is to transmit all necessary information in a way that's as simple and unintimidating as possible.

877 Timing is everything, and not just for insulin.

Choose your time carefully for speaking with your child's teacher. Trying to snag her attention when you're dropping off your child is a bad way to begin that relationship. Once class time starts, it's unfair to distract her from her primary responsibilities, even "just for a minute," and will guarantee a much-less-interested listener.

Much better plan: Call the school—before the academic year begins, if possible—and ask for a brief meeting with the teacher and the principal, so everybody can get on to the same page at a time when your child's welfare is the only topic of discussion.

878 That important ID bracelet...

If your child goes to school—even preschool—he needs a medical ID bracelet marked DIABETIC. Make sure he puts it on every day when he gets dressed. (You may have to remove a few links so that it will fit snugly and won't fall off.) You can find dozens of sources via a Google search.

879 ...And wristwatch.

As a mark of his being grown up enough to go to school, give your child an inexpensive watch and teach him to tell time. That way he can judge when to check his blood glucose, or when to have a snack.

880 Early puberty can cause blood-glucose problems.

In the past 60 years, puberty has come earlier and earlier. In the 1950s, it used to begin around the age of 13; now it often begins as early as nine or 10.

When you notice the beginning signs of puberty in your child, brace yourself for the inevitable: Your child's rapidly changing body and outrageous mood swings, caused by surging new hormones.

While all of these changes are true for all adolescents and their parents, they affect children with diabetes especially hard. Diabetic kids can experience wildly fluctuating blood sugars, so ask your pediatrician or endocrinologist to double their test-strip prescriptions so that your child can test every few hours, if necessary.

Be aware that puberty can also trigger type 2 diabetes in children who are seriously overweight. If your child is overweight, make sure that a blood-glucose test is part of every medical examination.

881 Teach your child body confidence.

Fact: Most children are not thin enough or beautiful enough to be magazine models, just as 99.9999% of adults are not.

Start teaching your child very early to be happy about her body, even if she's a little overweight. You do not want her to practice starvation as a dieting tool, even if all her friends are doing it.

Take the opportunity to show your daughter some of the legendary nude paintings by Rubens, Rembrandt, and Renoir to teach her that physical beauty and confidence come in all sizes and shapes. At the same time, encourage her to eat sensibly and be physically active.

Note: Although girls predominate, recent research shows that teenage boys have been going on starvation diets, too.

882 Make grocery shopping a learning experience...

Even preschoolers with diabetes can learn a lot about nutrition and making healthy choices during a trip to the supermarket. Involve them in making decisions—you can limit their options—and respect their food likes and dislikes. (Don't be surprised if their preferences change next month.)

Older children and adolescents can add to their skills, learning how to choose produce, meat, and fish, how to read and interpret labels, how to work within a food budget, and how each choice that is made impacts other choices.

883 ...And cooking, too.

Even young children can help in the kitchen—they love to! Preschoolers can help make salads and stir ingredients in a bowl. Older children can learn to use knives (carefully, under supervision!) and stovetops and ovens (ditto!). Consult with them on trying out new recipes, tweaking old favorites, and even creating new dishes—for example, starting with chicken, then adding uncommon and unique vegetables, herbs, and spices.

884 Try a mini triathlon.

Scale down a triathlon for your child. (It will still be exciting and pleasurable; remember to test blood glucose first and have a snack, if needed.)

Younger children can probably ride their bicycles up and down the street once, walk or run the same distance, and swim two laps freestyle in the back-yard pool. Teenagers can multiply these distances by five times, then 10.

You are the cheering section! Reward your child for finishing the triathlon—don't time kids until they ask you to. Considering their exertion, a small portion of ice cream is a wonderfully suitable reward.

885 Eat together.

Even if you're eating different foods for health or other reasons, sit down and face each other. It's a bonding time. Use mealtime as a be-together occasion, not an opportunity to criticize manners or scold for ignoring the "healthy stuff" on their plates. The supportive bonds you build over shared mealtimes will make it easier to suggest or enforce less-popular health directives later on.

886 How much slack can you cut your teen?

Physicians, psychologists, and diabetics can all testify: Going through puberty as a diabetic teen is infinitely more complicated than dealing with either situation alone. The mood swings and raging hormones of adolescence are multiplied, warped, and amplified by the mood swings and raging hormones of galloping blood-glucose levels, and the disease is a perfect setup for teenage risk-taking behavior.

As much as possible, help your teen keep social and personal identity issues separate from diabetic issues. Battles over blood glucose control and even some safety issues need to be seen by parents through the age-normal prisms of independence struggles and autonomy issues.

887 Plan now for those teen years.

Without putting a too Pollyanna-ish face on the situation, I think that parents whose young children are diagnosed with type 1 or type 2 diabetes are oddly lucky in one respect: They can establish habits, expectations, and influence from the child's early age, and this can be much easier than presenting new restrictions to a headstrong teen. The openness, respect, and authority you establish with your toddler or school-age child will assist you both greatly when he reaches his mid-teens.

888 The skin they're in can be more comfortable.

Your child's objections to being diabetic are based largely on the dietary restrictions and discomforts of the disease. Nothing else is really real to him, and future complications seem forever away, if he even believes they are possible.

Minimizing comfort complaints can make your child's diabetes much easier emotionally as well as physically. For dry skin, especially in winter, ordinary moisturizing lotions can help, but some children may need stronger remedies. Look for body lotions without alcohol (it's drying). Lotions that contain mineral oil are good, because of its properties as a moisture sealant. Ask your pharmacist or health-food store for Bag Balm, a cream developed for healing cows' udders, or buy it online. It also turns out to be fabulous for skiers' frostbitten and windburned faces, and many nurses have quietly used it for years to prevent bedsores on their patients. As Bag Balm has the consistency of petroleum jelly and a strong smell, give your child enough time for it to be absorbed and the smell to dissipate before getting dressed.

889 Don't let a label throw you—or them.

From nursery school until long past our teen years, a label can rankle and plow up all kinds of negative feelings.

Try to remember and instill in your child: Attitudes hold you back. Because some federal laws label diabetes as a "disability," diabetic children are entitled to special considerations in schools—everything from "shadow teachers" for children whose blood-glucose swings cause behavior problems to extra time and assistance when taking the SAT exams. More than any sensitive child, yours needs to learn that a label is "just a word, not a sentence."

890 We're from the government and we're here to help you.

The National Diabetes Education Program has information on assisting children with diabetes. Its Resources on Diabetes in Children and Adolescents offers a booklet titled "Helping the Student with Diabetes Succeed: A Guide for School Personnel." It's invaluable for parents, in order to know what educators and administrators should know. The booklet is free and is available from the NDEP website, NDEP.nih.gov.

Another arm of the federal government, the Department of Justice's Civil Rights Division, has details of the Americans with Disabilities Act and what to do about discrimination. Log on to Justice.gov/crt/disability-rights-section.

891 Don't be intimidated: Here's a good place to start.

If you've already Googled "diabetes," you've been swamped with way too much information. Don't be alarmed. The National Diabetes Information Clearinghouse—a service of the National Institute of Diabetes and Digestive and Kidney Diseases (NIDDK)—breaks a lot of data and resources into accessible chunks. They'll answer questions about diabetes by phone, fax, mail, and email; just remember to call between 8:30 a.m. and 5:00 p.m. Eastern Time, Monday through Friday.

The NIDDK offers booklets, brochures, and online information, copyright-free and on several reading levels. The website can also refer you to local health organizations. *Contact the NIDDK at...*

National Institute of Diabetes and Digestive and Kidney Diseases (NIDDK)

9000 Rockville Pike
Bethesda, MD 20892-3560
Phone: (800) 860-8747, (866) 569-1162 (TTY)
Fax: (301) 634-0716
Email: healthinfo@niddk.nih.gov
Website: NIDDK.nih.gov

892 Open wide and say "aaah."

Tooth and gum problems can be more prevalent in people with diabetes. Everyone's plaque buildup includes germs, but high blood glucose helps germs and bacteria flourish and multiply. That leads to bad breath and sore and swollen gums that bleed when you brush your teeth.

Children with diabetes can have tooth and gum problems more often if their blood glucose is poorly controlled. Check your child's smile regularly. Sore, bleeding gums are the first signs of periodontal (gum) disease, which can lead to infection in the gums and bone that holds the teeth. Infection may cause your child's gums to pull away from his teeth, and could even lead to premature bone loss. Regular flossing and brushing are a great help, and so is visiting the dentist twice a year.

893 Make sure your child's a "shoe-in."

Foot damage is a constant threat to people with diabetes, who may not feel blisters or injuries when they happen. Make sure your child always wears socks or stockings with her shoes or hard-backed slippers, to avoid blisters. Knee-high stockings or socks that are too tight at the top are also an invitation to problems because they restrict circulation.

Most importantly, check your child's shoes weekly to make sure that they still fit well. Make sure that a growth spurt isn't trapping your child's feet in suddenly-too-small shoes. Do your shoe-shopping at the end of the day, when your child's feet are their largest. And have your child break in new shoes by wearing them only for an hour or two a day for the first week. Sandals may be a better choice for the rest of the time.

894 Check your child's shoes every morning.

Everyone in Texas and the Southwest learns to check inside a shoe before putting it on—scorpions, spiders, and other nasty critters may have crawled into the warm, dark recess. But even in Saskatchewan or Duluth, checking inside your child's shoes before putting them on is a good habit to develop. Tiny toys, loose shoe tacks, or other sharp-edged hazards might be hiding, ready to injure your child's feet.

895 Don't push food on your kids.

Even toddlers and preschoolers are much better at gauging their appetites than their parents are. Your kids are more likely not to overeat if you let them serve themselves or if you serve them small portions and let them ask for more.

Urging them to take one more spoonful for Mommy/Daddy/Grandma and the whole darn extended family can lead to lifelong overeating and childhood obesity.

896 Make sure your pediatrician checks your child's blood pressure.

Pediatricians should be taking blood-pressure readings at every routine visit starting at age three. High blood pressure can start in children and do great damage before it is officially diagnosed or treated, and children with diabetes are especially vulnerable. Ask the doctor to check your child's blood pressure at the three-month checkups. (Children with diabetes should have three-month checkups rather than just one annual well visit.)

897 Have your child checked for gluten sensitivity.

Medical researchers now recommend that children with type 1 diabetes be tested for celiac disease, or gluten sensitivity. Celiac disease is a chronic immune genetic disorder that makes people unable to tolerate gluten, a protein found in wheat, rye, and barley. When they eat foods containing gluten, their immune systems respond by damaging the lining of the small intestine. As the damaged areas can't absorb nutrients properly, people with celiac disease become malnourished—no matter how much or how well they eat. Controlling your child's blood-glucose levels and nutritional intake will be much easier when you know whether she has a gluten sensitivity.

According to the Celiac Disease Foundation, the American Diabetes Association recommends screening children for celiac disease shortly after the diagnosis of type 1 diabetes.

898 Make your relationship healthy.

Having a child with diabetes means even more riding herd, questioning and checking, and striving for control. Confine that need for strict control to your child's diabetes. Maintaining a healthy relationship with your child demands a great deal of self-control and self-awareness on your part. If necessary, keep an actual private count of your positive interactions each day. Make sure that you're not just a police officer or a "measurer," but also a warm, safe, nurturing parent. If most of your conversations with your child are about restrictions or control, expect power struggles and resentment.

899 Don't punish your child for diabetes-related slips.

"Discipline" actually means "guidance." Punishing your child for anything relating to his diabetes makes the disease seem even more unfair. All kids sneak sweets; when yours does, too, receiving the same punishment as when he does something deliberate or defiant makes the disease even harder to bear.

Yes, the immediate results are worse for your child, but it's also true that kids forget and accidents happen. If you can, use diabetes-related slips as teaching moments rather than punishment occasions. Your getting angry can inspire equal and opposing anger, or hopelessness or guilt—or all of these emotions.

900 Your child is a separate person, and nobody's always perfect.

Two of the greatest stress-inducers in parents are (wrongly) seeing their children as extensions of themselves rather than as separate individuals, and (wrongly) seeing diabetes as a flaw or a failure. Before you laugh, ask yourself if you've ever uttered (or thought) the phrase, "How could a child of mine...?"

Diabetes is a physical condition, not a failure; your child's physiology does not reflect on your character or parenting—unless you're feeding your child junk food and letting him turn into a couch potato. Don't add guilt or pride to the already-stressful mix of emotions. Instead, use that energy to assist your child in finding coping strategies.

901 Are your child's slipups really a control struggle?

Occasionally forgetting his diabetes paraphernalia or insulin is one thing; habitual problems are something else. Make sure that the consequences of poor diabetes choices are appropriate to the "crime," and instruct your child in making better choices. Almost all children want more freedom. Taking some away when it's misused is much more effective—and instructive—than almost any other punishment.

902 A weekly "powwow" can be a great help.

Meeting with your diabetic child at the same time every week can be a great asset in problem solving and stress reduction. Ask your child to make a list of questions or problems, things that could or should be changed, and discuss them.

You can start your next weekly meeting by asking, "Well, how did we do on the things we discussed last week?"

903 Parents aren't always equal partners.

It can be hard to raise a diabetic child, and two-parent families don't always carry the load equally. Frequently, one parent carries more of the workload of the child's diabetes care; even more frequently, one parent carries more of the emotional load.

If you are the "less-burdened" parent, try to determine the scheduling limitations or discomfort with your child's illness—whatever keeps you less involved. If you are the parent who carries more of the load, do all you can to bring your spouse into the picture. Understanding that diabetes is not a failure or imperfection gives you greater insight into how it affects you, your spouse, and your child's life. Make efforts to minimize resentments so that you don't alienate your child from either parent.

904 Trade for treats.

Yes, the possible dire consequences may be the first thing that occurs to you when you catch your child sneaking sweets; but teaching your child to "trade for treats" is much more useful, in both the long term and the immediate moment.

Preteens aren't too young to learn how to compensate for treats. If he understands the balancing of food with insulin, and knows to tell an adult when he's hungry or having cravings both of you will be happier. You'll worry less about the possible consequences of his sneaking food, and he'll be more at ease knowing that he has a loving, caring backup.

Teach him early: Never, never sneak food without letting a parent or teacher know.

905 What to say to make everything worse.

Women are justifiably offended when someone suggests that their emotional state is due to monthly hormone fluctuations. Children with diabetes can often be just as offended when asked if their behavior is due to low blood sugar. Even when your intentions are good, asking that question is likely to infuriate a child who's already upset or angry—especially if you're right!

Rather than inquiring about blood-glucose level, consider offering your child a multiple choice: "Can I get you some turkey or a banana or something, as long as I'm up?" Phrased that way, a solution is possible without triggering emotional oversensitivity—or invalidating a real feeling by ascribing it to hormones. Your child could actually be justifiably angry without being hypoglycemic!

906 Don't call your child by his disease.

Let your child keep his personhood and not be labeled by his disease. Whenever possible, refer to him as "Joey, a boy with diabetes," rather than "a diabetic."

907 If possible, have your babysitter take a Red Cross course.

The best babysitter isn't just someone your child likes who's free on Saturday night. As your child needs special attention regarding when and what she eats, your babysitter needs some education about the symptoms of low blood sugar and how to treat it. You'll have to do much of this individual educating yourself.

For the general, nondiabetic babysitting issues, the American Red Cross has developed an excellent course in babysitting geared to teenagers, and your local chapter can tell you when this course is offered near you. Safe Sitter, Inc., is another organization that offers a babysitting course for children older than 11. Call (317) 596-5001 to see if there is a program near you, or go to SafeSitter.org.

908 Make your child a card-carrying person with diabetes.

Teaching your child to take ownership of her diabetes is vital. Who will be watching your child once she leaves your home? Joining the American Diabetes Association (Diabetes.org) and the Juvenile Diabetes Research Foundation (JDRF.org) makes great sense for anyone with diabetes in the family. Membership offers many benefits not listed in their pamphlets. Your child can read about diabetes in materials appropriate to her age level, making self-care easier and taking some of the burden off you, the parent.

909 School lunches as portable smorgasbords get eaten more.

Prepackaged lunch kits are available in combinations suitable for diabetic meal plans, but read the labels carefully. They're loaded with MSG, fat, sugar, and salt. More importantly, you can't supervise the quality of the ingredients.

Making your own lunch kits, using little plastic containers, lets you duplicate the appeal of the commercial packs—and still control what's going into the lunch. Cubes of grilled chicken or lowfat cheese, plus baby carrots, cherry tomatoes, and berries, each in its own small plastic tub, turns a nutritious lunch into a scavenger hunt. Opening each little case makes discovering the next treat fun, and having small quantities of many foods increases the likelihood that your child will eat enough of the right things.

910 Cover your child's health while traveling.

You may go on vacation, but your child's diabetes won't be put on hold. Check with your health insurance company to make sure you and your child will be covered whenever you travel. If not, look into a special insurance policy for your vacation.

Talk to your child's doctor before you leave, especially if you're going out of the country or even to another time zone; you'll need adjustments to her insulin or medication schedule. Also, make sure her shots are up to date, and provide her with emergency medical ID and information.

And always carry twice as much insulin or medication as your child would normally need for the time away. *Don't pack these items in your checked suitcase—put them in your carry-on bag!*

911 Plan for winter.

Children with diabetes need to do some extra planning for winter. The drier air can make or worsen skin problems and itches, and winter also brings more colds and other viruses.

Be forewarned: Illness stresses the body, so blood-glucose levels go up when your child is ill, making it more difficult to control his diabetes. Talk to your child's endocrinologist or pediatrician now about how to handle sick days.

912 Consider sewing solutions for children who wear pumps.

A needle and thread and a little creativity can make it easier for your child to wear an insulin pump. Even very young children are using insulin pumps now, but toddlers' clothes frequently don't have the belts and design features that allow the pump to be worn easily.

If your child resists the harness that comes with some pumps, make her a new undergarment: Sewing a 4"x4" square of cotton jersey (from an outgrown T-shirt) onto the back of her T-shirt creates a pouch that holds a pump easily. And her remodeled T-shirt needs no special laundering instructions. She can wear the shirt under other clothes. Putting the pouch in the back moves it out of her way but still leaves it accessible.

913 Believe that breakfast is the most important meal.

We've all heard that breakfast is the most important meal of the day. That's even more true for children with diabetes. Your child will need food for energy to start his day. Blood sugars may be low after not having eaten all night, and a good breakfast of foods on his meal plan will help him feel better and concentrate.

One note: An egg would seem to be an obvious protein choice, but the Harvard School of Public Health website (HSPH.harvard.edu) advises people with diabetes to have no more than three egg yolks per week. Consider cooking liquid egg substitute or egg whites, or serving lowfat cottage cheese or string cheese, Canadian bacon or lean ham, sliced turkey or lean roast beef, water-pack tuna, a handful of unsalted nuts, or peanut butter.

914 Be safe to talk to.

Children need someone safe to talk to about their diabetes and how it makes them feel. Difficult as it may be, separating your feelings from just listening is vital. As a beloved adult, you are not only a source of information, you also need to be a safe harbor for frustrations and fears about the repercussions of ignoring diabetes. Don't let your responses make your child equate a high blood-glucose level with shame and blame—he needs you to be safe to talk to…about anything.

915 Don't neglect your other children.

This should be obvious. (Nobody said it was easy!) 'Nuff said.

CHAPTER 8

Tips for Diabetics Who Live Alone

All the tips in this chapter relate to feeling—and being—less vulnerable and less prone to accidents even though you have diabetes and live alone. When you feel safe, you are less stressed. As a result, your blood-glucose levels stay more even.

916 Celebrate your singleness.

Attitude can be everything, especially when you're the only one in the house. Yes, living alone has the drawback of occasional loneliness. It also has the advantage of enormous privacy. You can run around the house in a moose mask all day if you like (and if the curtains are closed). You can watch TV till 2:00 a.m., grill a hamburger for breakfast, or do yoga in the living room in the nude. Since everything in life is a trade-off, focus on what you gain by your single lifestyle, rather than griping about what you may feel is lacking in any one moment.

917 Don't leave home without it.

Don't even think of going out of town without giving a trusted friend a copy of your itinerary. Every single person should do this, diabetic or not. If you haven't alerted people to expect you at a certain place at a certain time, how could they know if something were amiss? Following this tip assists you and gives peace of mind to everyone who cares about you.

918 Is that your watch vibrating, or are you just glad to see me?

Self-care for your diabetes is your responsibility, but living alone makes it that much more important to remember all the checkpoints in your day.

A fabulous but subtle helper is a vibrating watch: Rather than sounding an alarm, it gives the wearer an unmistakable (but silent) wake-up or reminder. Unless you're holding someone's hand at the moment, the shaking is your own private alert. Originally created for people with hearing loss, a vibrating watch can keep us on schedule, too. Go online and Google "vibrating watch." You'll find an extensive assortment of brands and prices to choose from.

919 Give yourself a free space.

One of the toughest aspects of living alone is misplacing something vital. You pretty much need your glasses to find your glasses, and where are you if you can't find your car keys?

Designate a spot in your home—the bottom of your underwear drawer, a kitchen shelf, a table in your front hallway, wherever—to be the "home base" for possessions that you absolutely can't lose. When your glasses aren't on the bridge of your nose, they'll be in your "spot." When your car keys aren't in your hand or in the ignition, they'll be in your "spot." Be as obsessive and compulsive about this as possible—you'll never be sorry.

You may want another space—near your bed?—for your glucose meter, test strips, lancet, and glucose tablets.

920 Know your neighbors.

Because you live alone, get to know your neighbors. Be aware of who their family and relatives are, and get an idea of their normal schedules. Preventing burglary next door may keep you safe as well.

Also, tell your neighbors that you have diabetes, and ask them to ring your doorbell or phone you if they don't see you at the usual times.

921 Knock three times.

If you live in an apartment or town house where you share a common wall with a neighbor, arrange a signal in case you need help. You can knock on the wall, blow a whistle, or find another audible sign in case your blood glucose is dropping and you can't use your phone.

922 Take your diabetes to sea.

Who says controlling your diabetes can't be fun? Go online and see how many different cruises are offered for people with diabetes. Not only will you be aboard with like-minded cruising companions, you'd also be catered to by chefs cooking for your special needs.

And check with your tax consultant. Some special-for-diabetics cruises also offer educational seminars aboard. See whether you can deduct a portion of the cost of your cruise, since it is medically oriented.

923 You know how to whistle, don't you?

Put a whistle on your keychain, and consider wearing one on a ribbon or chain around your neck—outside and inside your home. If you're outside and anyone tries to bother you, blowing that whistle makes you too much audible trouble to mess with. And just as important, wearing your whistle inside your home lets you summon help—sometimes even through apartment walls! It doesn't have to be an expensive stainless-steel coach's whistle—often plastic dime-store whistles can emit loud, piercing shrieks, and are made in bright neon colors that are easy to spot at the bottom of a handbag.

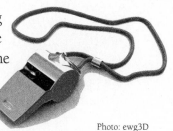

Photo: ewg3D

924 Dawdle over dinner.

Too many people who live alone race through their meals in front of the TV. Make your dinner last at least 45 minutes. When you slow down, some wonderful things happen...

- **You turn eating into dining, a pleasurable experience.**
- **You give your body the opportunity to start feeling full,** a process that takes 20 to 30 minutes.
- **...which means there's less chance that you'll mindlessly overeat.**

Instead of eating while watching TV, listen to music. Slow Baroque and classical music are especially good.

925 Use a buddy system.

You should have someone to check in with every morning. Your buddy doesn't have to have diabetes; anyone who lives alone and might need help will benefit from this arrangement, and so will you.

Your call can be brief: "Hi, it's me. Are you OK? I'm OK. Do you need anything?"

What counts is that you and your friend have made sure that each of you is alive and well.

926 Don't be too proud to use a cane.

Many people use a cane in the winter to navigate snowy and icy streets, only because they can't afford to risk falling and breaking a bone. If you have diabetes, your balance may be compromised, so this tip is even more important for you. One of my neighbors, who does not have diabetes, took a fall on New

Year's Day and wound up with a compound shoulder fracture that necessitated hours of surgery and months of physical therapy!

Use a cane that's beautiful so that it will give you pleasure. Mine has a brass bulldog's head, and I'm looking for others so that they become fashion statements. If you live alone where there is a lot of snow and ice, ski poles and/or crampons for your shoes may help you avoid a fall. One Boston friend attaches Yaktrax™ to the bottom of her boots.

927 Raising cane I: Get the right support.

Do you need a cane occasionally, for a little extra support? Then any cane that feels comfortable should do just fine.

But if you need a heavy-duty cane that can support a person who weighs 500 pounds, you should really try it before you buy it—or make sure you can return it.

Very heavy bariatric canes, which can support someone who weighs 700 pounds, are made of 1" steel tubing to bear the weight safely.

928 Raising cane II: You need at least two.

Because you live alone and never know when you may experience mobility problems, you should have at least two canes—one by your bed, one by your front door. Always use your bedside cane for those middle-of-the-night bathroom excursions. If you feel even a little bit shaky, this tip is mandatory, as it beats a possible fall.

Your front-door cane is for bad weather, for stability, for flagging down a bus driver, and for getting a seat on that bus, if it's crowded.

929 Raising cane III: You may need a quad cane.

Quad canes have four tips at the bottom for greater stability. They can be helpful if you need more support than a single tip provides.

Even greater support is provided with a quad cane that has four sharp steel prongs at the bottom, released by a spring. This is my choice for navigating winter ice and snow.

930 Raising cane IV: Your cane has other uses.

Your cane can substitute for a stepladder, which is certainly more risky.

If you have to put something on a high shelf, put it at the front of the shelf, then use the handle of the cane to push the item back. To get it down, hook the handle of the cane around it and pull it carefully toward you (or buy a long-armed grabber to help you).

And, obviously, canes are also great for reaching lost objects under furniture. They can also save you from getting down on your hands and knees.

931 Maybe you shouldn't lock up.

Admittedly, this advice is debatable. It depends on how safe your home and neighborhood are. It comes from a friend who has severe diabetes and who averages two or three trips to the emergency room every year. While he is glad that he's been rescued in time, he has gotten tired of EMS technicians breaking down his door to reach him.

If you feel safe in your home or apartment, keep your door unlocked when you go to sleep. If you need an ambulance for an emergency, EMS personnel won't have to break down your door—and then leave it open for potential burglars to wreak havoc.

932 Don't be shy.

If you live in an apartment, let your building staff know that you have diabetes and what your schedule is.

Leave standing instructions that if they don't see you by a certain time every morning, to ring your doorbell and—if there is no answer—to call 911.

And please tip them generously at holiday time!

933 Give your inner-circle friends permission.

Many people feel "hesitant to get involved," and they step away from situations because "It's not my place," or "I'm sure somebody will handle it." You don't need to have your condition "outed" if your diabetes is not common knowledge, but having an emergency contact list and giving it to trusted friends might save you lots of grief.

934 Carry, post, and share a contact list in case of emergency.

Keep the names and phone numbers in your wallet of geographically close friends who agree to be contacted in an emergency situation. Post a larger version of this list on your refrigerator, and share it with family and distant close friends.

When my friend sounded slow and disoriented on the phone, I called her neighbor—3,000 miles away. The neighbor went to check on her, and her blood glucose was so low that she was sliding into diabetic shock. Make sure you have shared a very local contact—even the doorman of your building—so that someone could come to your aid if you needed it.

935 Bathroom smarts I: Get the right grab rails.

Install heavy-duty grab rails by the bathtub. Make sure they will bear *at least 100 pounds more than your weight*; anything less is risky.

936 Bathroom smarts II: Create a skidproof tub.

Cover your tub with attractive adhesive motifs. Choose grippers that are as large as possible so that your feet will fit completely on them.

937 Bathroom smarts III: Have the right phone.

Cordless phones are usually the first phones people think of because they are so portable. But for the bathroom (and bedside), I recommend a phone that is directly connected to the circuitry because they will usually work even during power failures. In fact, during the Great Blackout of August 14, 2003, only my bedroom phone, which was hard-wired into the circuitry, worked. The five or six cordless and cell phones in different parts of the apartment were completely nonfunctioning!

938 Use your privacy to create new habits.

Habits often make us what we are. In fact, longtime ingrained habits are likely what makes controlling blood-glucose levels so difficult. But behavior experts say that creating a new habit can be done in just 28 days—that's less than a month!

So, since one of the joys of living alone is the privacy, use it! Put up big signs in the kitchen, or by the TV, reminding yourself of your new goals. And make some healthier new habits that will improve your life.

939 Outwit the portion-control marketers.

Almost everything you buy is sized wrong: Bottles, bags, boxes almost always contain at least two portions—usually more. Make unpacking your groceries a two-step process. Before putting away your purchases, break them down into portion-sized servings. Zipper-seal plastic storage and freezer bags make this very easy to do, so that grabbing a measured portion becomes effortless. It's the simplest way not to "just eat the broken chips" or "just finish the carton" or "polish off the rest of the bottle."

940 A cookbook for single people with diabetes.

The advantage of cooking for yourself is that you know the purity and quality of the ingredients that go into your meals. You know what went into what's going on your plate. A book by two registered dietitians, Kathleen Stanley and

Connie Crawley, offers more than 100 recipes for breakfasts, lunches, dinners and snacks for people with diabetes who are cooking single portions. *Quick & Easy Diabetic Recipes for One* is available at most brick-and-mortar and online bookstores, or through the American Diabetes Association.

941 Prepare ahead for the urge to grab something.

Being alone in the house, with nothing tasty and permissible *and* ready to eat, is almost a slam-dunk setup to grab something quick-and-easy—and off your eating plan. You can avoid this pitfall by doing a little preparation at a time when you're well fed and unhurried. Grill and wrap up a chicken breast, cut and clean some veggies…and you'll always have something immediately grabbable and satisfying. Even a can of chickpeas provides a complete protein with complex carbohydrates plus lots of chewing satisfaction. Add garlic, chili powder, or herbs for an extra spark of taste.

942 Be a card-carrying person with diabetes.

What if you were ever unable to speak for yourself? Wearing a medical ID bracelet and carrying a card in your wallet next to your driver's license is more than smart, it's vital. Your card should list data like your blood type (if you know it), whether you wear eyeglasses or contact lenses, and the names of your doctors. If your commuter train got derailed or a truck ran a light and plowed into your car, giving emergency personnel as much information as possible about your body will let them save valuable time and get you better care. (See Tip 420 and 421 for more information on IDing yourself.)

943 Cell phones were invented just for you.

"I've fallen and I can't get up" became a cliché because it's true so often—and not just for senior citizens. Living alone means nobody else is there, and the flip side (freedom and peace) is no help if you need it. Today's size, affordability, and availability of cell phones means that living alone isn't as dangerous anymore. A little device half the size and weight of your hand can fit in any pocket and follow you from room to room in your house. If you don't already have a cell phone, get one now.

944 Do you need another alarm system?

A number of companies sell medical-alarm systems that can be very handy if you have diabetes or a chronic disease. You wear an electronic pendant on a cord around your neck, and if you have an emergency, you press the button.

This activates a two-way system to call the monitoring center. You don't have to be able to reach your phone, and you may not have to speak into the pendant in some systems. Someone from the center will contact you immediately, 24 hours a day, and will then phone a designated friend or relative and the Emergency Medical Service, if necessary.

The cost seems to be pretty standard, with most of the companies charging approximately $30 per month. Comparison-shop to find the medical-alarm system that matches your needs.

945 Stay motivated.

Living alone means it's often hard to stay motivated about blood-glucose control, keeping your spirits up during downturns in life events, and other problems. Keep pets, pictures of loved ones, or even portraits or photos of heroes or heroines around in full view. They can serve as reminders of love and courage during bad or just lonely times. Take strength from the knowledge that others depend on you to do the right thing, and if nobody currently does, then motivate yourself with the knowledge that you're behaving in ways that would make your heroes proud of you.

946 Take advantage of high-tech helpers.

"I forgot" just isn't an excuse that holds water anymore, ever since PDAs and watches began including health-tracking software. These gadgets have become affordable and stylish, and free software is now available to track all aspects of diabetes management from the palm of your hand. And ladies, if you're looking for a gift for a guy with diabetes, gadgets with bells and whistles can make even self-testing fun!

947 You deserve a fire extinguisher all your own.

Living alone means being the strongest link in your own chain—but also the weakest. Be prepared to handle any situation on your own by investing in and maintaining the equipment you might need in an emergency. Put a small fire extinguisher in your kitchen and a second one in your bedroom. Change the batteries in your smoke alarm twice a year and replace your carbon monoxide detector every five years.

948 Prepare to take on mother nature single-handedly.

If you live in an area prone to earthquakes, tornadoes, or ice storms, build a preparedness kit with a flashlight, some cash in case the ATMs are down, sneakers, deck shoes, or lightweight hiking boots, a Mylar blanket in case the heat goes off, extra socks and gloves, and a spare pair of glasses. More importantly, you should also include at least three days' worth of provisions and medications so you'll be able to get along until rescue workers can reach you or power is restored.

949 Keep a stash of emergency supplies.

Between blizzards and hurricanes and anything else that might cause power blackouts, you must keep emergency supplies on hand, especially if you live alone.

Besides the extra drugs and equipment mentioned in Chapter 1, you should have extra lightbulbs, several flashlights, and lots of extra batteries, a couple of transistor radios (one may fade out after a week of continuous use), a first-aid kit, at least five gallons of water, and lots of candles with sturdy candle-holders and matches.

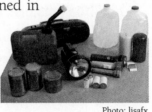

Photo: lisafx

Also a week's supply of canned food that you can eat cold in an emergency.

My favorites are mostly 100% protein: Chicken breast, salmon, and tuna, but I also include some canned ravioli and chili, in case I need some carbohydrates. *Make sure you have a hand-operated can opener so that you can get at this food during a power failure!*

950 Living alone safely with "Bruno."

Living alone means peace and quiet whenever you want it, but you might not want strangers to know that it's just you behind the front door. Consider posting a second name on your mailbox, something that sounds tough-but-not-made-up macho. That way, deliverymen and strangers casing your home will have to speculate on dealing with you *and* "Bruno McCormick"—not just you alone.

951 Licensed contractors are more than worth it.

Living alone means never hiring an unlicensed contractor to work in or even outside your home—even if your best friend swears by him. Contractors' licenses are overseen by local or state boards (depending on your municipality), which prefer to discipline their own miscreants from within. Hiring unlicensed people to do repairs or chores might seem cheaper, but your risks are higher—and not just financially.

952 Set up cheap and cheerful early warnings.

If you have a dog to wake you up if there are strange nighttime noises, it's a wonderful burglar alarm. And unless you have a cat, hanging inexpensive glass wind chimes on your doorknob when you lock up for the night can be a lifesaver: If you hear them tinkling in the night, someone is trying to open your door. Little bells would work as well unless, again, you have a cat that would love to bat them around playfully.

Hearing the wind chimes jingle gives you time to dial 911 on your bedside phone. You *do* have a phone at your bedside, right? And some people go as far as putting bottles or other breakables on their windowsills, which makes a lot of clatter if someone tries to break in.

953 Don't dismiss your instincts.

Whenever you feel uneasy being alone, trust your instincts.

One crime-prevention expert put it best: "We are the only mammal on the planet that dismisses our instinct most of the time," usually out of concern about overdramatizing or being seen as hysterical or paranoid.

If you sense you're being followed, go inside a business or store and ask to call 911. If someone is approaching you, cross the street. If you are cornered, scream and holler and call attention to yourself—be more trouble to bother than you're worth.

954 Keep a flashlight in or near your bed.

There are lots of reasons to keep this handy little tool nearby: To check on suspicious noises, to light your way during a power failure, even to locate something that's rolled under your bed. Having a flashlight close by could be especially important if you feel low and want to test your blood glucose, but the power is out.

955 Goof-proof your home.

Do a safety check of your home for potential hazards: Rugs that can slide and trip you, slippery bathtubs, beautifully waxed floors. All of these can cause leg or hip fractures.

Your local Visiting Nurse Service may offer help from occupational therapists who can advise you on safety issues.

956 Protect yourself from sharp-edged furniture...

Why do we fall against sharp-edged furniture, especially at 3:00 a.m. when our blood glucose is dropping? Because it's there!

How to prevent or minimize those black-and-blue marks and potential fractures? Pad everything! Use folded towels or movers' pads. Color coordination is an attractive plus, but your real goal is protecting yourself from injury.

957 …And protect yourself from doorknobs, too.

Even though doorknobs are smooth, you can still do yourself major damage if you fall against one in a hypoglycemic swoon because they are just the right height for you to hit your head against them as you go down for the count.

For an easy fix, cover the offending doorknob with bubble wrap and secure it with rubber bands. For a more color-coordinated fix, cover that with an attractive washcloth.

958 Post medical emergency information in all the right places.

Put this information on two sheets of paper on which you have drawn a big red border and title it MEDICAL EMERGENCY INFORMATION. Write the same information on each of them…your name, medical problems, the drugs you are taking, any allergies or drug reactions, the name and phone number of your contact person, and your blood type, if you know it.

Stick one of the pages onto the inside of your front door with a magnet, and display the other prominently on your refrigerator door.

959 Don't miss a step.

If your fuse box or circuit breakers are in your basement, paint the edge of every step with luminous white or Day-Glo paint. Then, if your power goes out, you'll manage to get safely down the basement stairs to change the fuse or reset the circuit breakers. And always take a flashlight!

960 Better balance, fewer falls.

Excluding hypoglycemia, most falls are caused by age-related problems: Arthritis, vision problems, drugs that cause dizziness or decreased alertness.

Gait and balance problems cause most major falls, so take these easy tests…

•**Walk heel-to-toe with one foot directly in front of the other.** Are you off-balance?

•**Stand on one leg for at least 20 seconds.** Repeat with the other leg. Are you off-balance? Any differences between your legs?

•**Sit in a chair without arms.** Rise, walk forward 10 feet, turn quickly, walk back, and sit. If this test takes you more than 14 seconds, you may be at risk for falling.

•**Discuss these results with your doctor.** Physical therapy may help.

961 Vitamin D can prevent or minimize falls.

According to a February 2008 article in *Pharmacotherapy*, there is a "statistically significant positive relationship between vitamin D supplementation with either cholecalciferol 700 IU per day or greater, or ergocalciferol 800 IU per day or greater, and decreased risk of falls."

As safe daily doses of these two forms of vitamin D range up to 1,100 IU, vitamin D seems like a good idea, especially for us Northerners who don't often make enough vitamin D in our own bodies from sun exposure.

962 Don't wait for prince(ss) charming.

What are you waiting for? Living alone means never having to ask, "Where's my bathrobe?" Waiting for somebody else to come along and give you a life is a double waste. You're missing weeks and years of private joys and adventures, and resenting some amorphous providence for not delivering on your own expectations. Making your own life as you go through it chapter by chapter is not only smarter and more efficient, but also taking responsibility for your attitudes and adventures puts *you* in charge.

CHAPTER 9

Solving Special Problems

GENERAL
---

963 How much of a warning do you need?

Many people got a warning recently, if they and their doctors were wise enough to heed it. "Prediabetes" refers to levels of blood glucose higher than normal, but less than the cutoff for a diagnosis of diabetes. The American Diabetes Association has recommended lower guideline numbers defining prediabetes; the idea is to head diabetes off at the pass before it's full-blown. If your fasting blood glucose reads between 100 and 125, or your nonfasting is 140 or higher at any time of the day, your doctor should share your lab results with you immediately. Putting small changes into your lifestyle now could make the difference between developing diabetes or not.

964 Keep it level.

Some people mistakenly imagine that type 2 (insulin resistant) diabetes is somehow less serious than type 1 (insulin dependent) diabetes. Not so, and both require very close monitoring of blood glucose levels. Type 2s have a very high risk of heart disease and stroke. Even if your doctor prescribes oral medication rather than insulin injections, both types of diabetes can lead to problems like kidney and eye disease, nerve damage, and dementia. Keeping your blood glucose level between 90 and 130 before meals, and lower than 180 two hours after meals, is important no matter what diabetes medications you take. (Seniors can have higher blood glucose levels; check with your doctor.)

965 It's a closed system.

Realize that your body is a closed system: It's all connected. Your control of your diabetes—or the lack of it—will have a profound effect on your heart and blood vessels, your eyes, your kidneys, your feet, your nervous system—even your skin and your sex life.

966 Mine the Internet for support and information.

The amount of responsible diabetes information available on the Internet is truly amazing and heartening. Use google.com to refine your search and narrow it further by linking two or three key words instead of just one—e.g., diabetes+eye problems.

I especially like the website of the 24 medical boards that are members of the American Board of Medical Specialties (www.abms.org links to individual specialty boards) and the InDependent Diabetes Trust (www.IDDT.org) for a British and European perspective on diabetes. For less technical information, check the American Diabetes Association website (Diabetes.org) and Bottom Line's Diabetes Resource Center (BottomLineInc.com/resource-center/diabetes).

967 Are you married to a diabetic lifestyle?

The diabetes you prevent can be not only yours, but also your significant other's. In a study done at the Royal London Hospital, and published in *Diabetes Care* in 2003, researchers checked diabetes warning signals—weight, blood pressure, exercise habits, food choices, and smoking—and discovered that if one spouse already had diabetes, the other had significantly higher risk. Although diabetes isn't contagious, a "diabetes lifestyle" can be. The researchers recommended getting screened if your partner has diabetes, and making walking dates together to share the time and the benefits of regular exercise.

968 Diabetes ain't doom, and it ain't depression, either.

Just like taking responsibility for managing your own blood-glucose levels, to a very large degree, you can also manage your own happiness levels. According to happiness researcher Sonja Lyubomirsky, PhD, of the University of California, Riverside, about 40% of our happiness is influenced by what we deliberately do to make ourselves happy.

Her suggestions? Look for what's right—rather than what's wrong—with a day, a person, or a situation. Be grateful and kind as often as possible. Create a rich and full social and friendship network. And make sure that you get enough rest, quiet, and solitude for balance.

969 Prevention beats treatment.

As in all areas of life, prevention makes more sense than treatment. Prevention means intervening early to change and correct situations before they become problems. Prevention is much easier, faster, and cheaper. It's a much smarter move!

PAIN RELIEF

---

970 Realize the bright side of pain.

Amazingly, there is one. Pain is a symptom that something is not right and needs attention and care. When you can't feel pain immediately, as in some forms of neuropathy, you can suffer unknowingly, and your body might experience major damage. That said, you'll find the following resources useful…

971 Find the right doctor for your pain.

Every large hospital has many pain-relief doctors. Some specialize in pain caused by orthopedic problems; some specialize in pain caused by cancer; some treat general pain. Go to the hospital's website and filter the doctors in the pain-relief department by the doctor's subspecialty, the languages spoken, and whether the doctor is accepting new patients. "Auditioning" the candidates' qualifications will make it a better match for you.

972 Even if you hurt, you're not alone.

The American Chronic Pain Association offers peer support and education in pain management skills to people with pain, family and friends, and health care professionals. Today several hundred ACPA support groups meet across the US and in Canada, Great Britain, and many other countries. The ACPA's unique materials are a primary resource for individuals seeking to improve the quality of their lives and for the professionals who help them. To find a support group near you, visit their webite theacpa.org/Support-Groups or call 800-533-3231.

973 Rub out your pain?

Before taking more expensive and more invasive steps, see if massage therapy offers some pain relief. The book *Trigger Point Therapy for Myofascial Pain* by Donna Finando LAc (Licensed Acupuncturist), LMT (Licensed Massage Therapist) and Steven Finando, PhD, LAc, offers massage and pressure techniques to ease pain and prevent its return. Amazon.com, BarnesandNoble.com and other booksellers also offer many other massage-therapy books.

974 Know that pain can cause increased blood-glucose readings.

According to an American Diabetes Association report dated August 17, 2015, both short-term and long-term pain can cause increased blood-glucose readings. That's because pain releases adrenaline, which, in turn, raises blood glucose. It's not your fault—just increase your diabetes medications.

975 Hail the lowly heating pad!

Heat may be all you need to relieve pain. Use a heating pad for up to one hour where it hurts, remove it for one-half hour, and repeat. If you get no relief after one day, you may need a stronger localized medication, like a lidocaine patch or lidocaine cream.

HYPOGLYCEMIA

---

976 Don't leave home without it.

Keep glucose gel or tablets or a roll of Lifesavers in your purse or briefcase, another stash in your desk, and still another under your pillow. When your blood-glucose level drops like a rock, you'll want this help within easy reach. A tube of glucose gel contains up to 24 grams of carbohydrate, depending on how much you can actually get into your mouth and swallow. One glucose tablet contains 4 grams of carbohydrate, so you'll want to take four or five of them to counter hypoglycemia.

977 Have a sliding scale.

Discuss with your diabetes specialist whether it's appropriate to have one plan if your blood glucose drops to around 55-60 and another more radical plan if it drops to 40-50—or whether "more of the same" is right for you.

978 Glucagon: Not if you live alone.

Glucagon is a wonderful first-response remedy for hypoglycemia, but it is useless if you live alone or are alone. If your blood glucose sinks so low that you need a rapid-response glucose injection, you're not going to have the brain power or coordination to give yourself an injection, or to call a neighbor you've trained to do it. The only thing you can do to protect yourself is to test your blood glucose if you even suspect it is dropping, and to devour a tube of glucose gel or four or five glucose tablets if your test result is 60 or lower.

979 Be aware of glucagon's short shelf life.

Glucagon remains potent for only 18 months. Check the expiration date when you pick up your glucagon kit at the pharmacy. Make a note in your daybook for December 31: "Glucagon expires (date)—get a new one" and transfer it to the appropriate month of next year's daybook, or put the expiration reminder into your electronic calendar for the proper date to refill.

980 If you must choose.

It's far from the ideal solution, but if you must choose between high and low blood-glucose levels, you will damage your body much less by having a blood glucose over 300 than a blood glucose under 50 for one hour.

981 Be a safe driver.

There are countless horror stories about people with diabetes causing car accidents because of a hypoglycemic attack—probably about as many as people suffering heart attacks at the wheel and crashing.

To be safe, *always* test your blood glucose just before you pick up your car keys—even if it means testing three or four more times a day. And if you suddenly feel dizzy when you're at the wheel, pull off the road for a few minutes and gobble a tube of glucose gel or a few glucose tablets.

982 Checking for hypoglycemia? Test here only.

Most of the time, it's OK to use blood from your arm, thigh, or calf. But when you are checking for possible hypoglycemia, only finger sticks are accurate. It's not unusual to get a blood-glucose reading of 70 from your forearm, but only 40 from your finger.

983 After you've corrected for hypoglycemia.

After you've consumed glucose in some form or fruit juice to raise your blood sugar, wait one-half hour, then test again. In rare instances, you may not have consumed enough glucose and may need to take more. You should bring your blood glucose up to around 100 to be safe after hypoglycemia.

984 Tight control may increase the risk of severe hypoglycemia.

People with type 1 diabetes who are controlling their diabetes intensively are more likely to experience severe hypoglycemia than people with diabetes who are using ordinary control.

If this profile fits you and you experience hypoglycemia as often as once a week, ask your doctor to evaluate your drugs and dosages.

985 Pattern recognition can help you prevent hypoglycemia.

You test your blood glucose first thing every morning and keep a record of the numbers. What if your fasting numbers are between 55 and 100 90% of the time? *There are several things you can do…*

• **Call your diabetes doctor** and ask to have your medication adjusted.

• **Eat a slightly bigger breakfast,** but go easy on the carbohydrates.

• **If you've been taking insulin for many years and are a very compliant patient,** you may want to reduce your fast-acting insulin by one unit and record your new fasting blood sugars. They should rise to around 120.

• **Then call your diabetes doctor to report what you've done.**

986 Is it a stroke—or hypoglycemia?

The symptoms may look and feel the same: Confusion, slurred speech, trouble walking. *But* if you're under 40 years of age, it's more likely that you have hypoglycemia. The fastest and easiest way to check is to eat or drink glucose or fructose—you don't want to wait for sugar to metabolize—and lie down for 15 to 20 minutes.

Then check your blood glucose. Is it over 80 now? Have your symptoms decreased? You've probably just had a hypoglycemic episode, but if you're unsure, call 911.

987 Sometimes you can tell when hypoglycemia is coming on.

After being on insulin for 30 years, I can usually tell when a hypoglycemic episode is on the way. I've been outside running errands, and suddenly there it is: The scary feeling that if I can't get home in a couple of minutes, I'll fall down in the street. (If this happens to you and you've forgotten your to-go glucose, stop at a drugstore or convenience store and buy a small pack of jelly beans to protect yourself from hypoglycemia.)

And when I get home and test my blood glucose, it's in the low 40s! I eat something immediately and am glad I got home in time.

988 Know how quickly your blood glucose drops.

Are you just relaxing or working at your desk? Your blood glucose may drop only 20 to 30 points in an hour—lots of time to wait and test before your next meal.

But if you're walking around or doing even light exercise, your blood glucose can drop as much as 50 points in an hour, which can cause hypoglycemia risk. Then you'll want to eat earlier than usual.

SICK DAYS

989 Sick days require at least two plans.

Most books and magazines for people with diabetes urge us to have a plan for sick days. But I think we need at least two. We need one plan for fever and colds, but when we can eat normally; another when we can't keep any food down and have diarrhea. When you are "ejecting from both ends," you will need to take less insulin and drink liquids like Gatorade that will restore your electrolytes.

Set up these plans *now*. When you're really sick, you're not thinking clearly enough to do it.

990 Avoid dehydration.

Dehydration is a serious problem faced by people with diabetes when they get sick. Among the symptoms that increase the risk of dehydration are fever, vomiting, and diarrhea. Drink at least two quarts of water every day (especially when you're sick)—more if you can stand it.

Ask your doctor whether you need to increase your salt intake to keep your electrolytes in balance, as you may have lost sodium as well as fluids.

991 Sick days are like high-stress days.

Your body's response to illness is very similar to its response to stress. Your blood-glucose level can rise 100 to 200 points overnight—and it's not because you over ate.

Sick days are just a fact of life—for some people with diabetes, perhaps a little more frequent in our lives. But now you have plans in place to deal with both high-stress days and sick days.

992 Sick days mean more insulin.

You will probably have to use more insulin when you are sick. Discuss with your doctor how many more units of insulin—and which types—for every 50 points of increased blood glucose. And check in with your doctor every day that you are sick; it may save a trip to the emergency room.

THINKING CLEARLY

993 "Brain fog" and how to lift it.

Often "brain fog" is caused by high blood-glucose levels—over 200 for at least a week. High sugars actually thicken the blood. The farther from the heart and the smaller and narrower the blood vessel, the more slowly the blood will move and the less efficiently it will deliver oxygen and remove wastes from the tissues. The brain is so sensitive to being well nourished and cleaned of wastes that it is the *most affected part of the body when blood sugars skyrocket.*

If you can keep your blood sugars down to normal levels for at least a week, you will definitely notice the difference in your thinking!

994 "Brain fog" can also be caused by hypoglycemia.

Paradoxically, "brain fog" can also be caused by dropping blood glucose. If your thinking starts to get fuzzy, check your blood sugar first.

995 More about memory impairment.

Check your carbohydrate intake before you blame Alzheimer's. Researchers at UCLA reported in the May 17, 2012, issue of *Forbes* magazine that just six weeks of feeding laboratory animals a fructose solution (designed to mimic people drinking soda) created dulled reactions. The rats that consumed the fructose solution were slower navigating a maze and their brains showed a decline in memory.

This study confirms an earlier one published in *Diabetes Care* in August 2003, in which the goal was to determine the impact of rapid carbohydrate consumption on human memory. It found that eating as little as 50 grams of quickly absorbed carbohydrate (one-half bagel and white grape juice) produced significant memory deficits in people with type 2 diabetes.

996 Soda is bad for your brain, but diet soda may be, too.

Both kinds of soda correlated with faster brain aging. While more research needs to be done, a recent Boston University study reported in *Stroke* found that people who drank diet soda every day were three times as likely to develop stroke and dementia compared with people who did not drink diet soda.

EYES

---

997 Get on the grid.

The Amsler grid is a simple visual test—a piece of graph paper you can get from your eye doctor or download from the Internet. It has black lines about ¼" apart with a big black dot right in the center.

The Amsler grid is a quick, easy test that shows you whether you have macular degeneration, even in its earliest stages. With normal retinal vision, you see all the lines at right angles, with the black dot in the center. But patients who have macular degeneration will see wavy lines and possibly blank areas.

Test yourself with the Amsler grid *at least once a week*, and call your eye doctor *immediately* if you find any changes.

How to use the Amsler Grid:

Wear your reading glasses, if you normally use them and sit about 14 inches away from the screen.

Cover the left eye.

With the right eye, focus on the dark dot in the center of the grid.

While looking at this dot, you still should be aware of the lines of the grid. Notice if any of the lines are distorted or broken or if there are blurred areas.

Now, cover the right eye and repeat the test.

If you notice any blurred, wavy, or missing lines, contact your ophthalmologist as soon as possible.

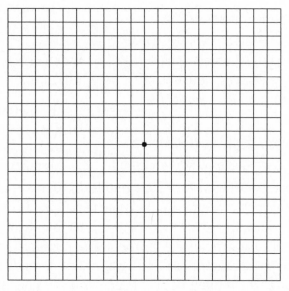

Remember that it is a "gross" test and may not catch early vision loss. You should see your eye doctor every year for a complete eye examination.

998 Wear your shades…let 'em call you star.

Eye problems are much more prevalent among people who have had diabetes for a while. The quickest, easiest way to head off forming cataracts is to wear sunglasses in bright sunlight to forestall the lens of the eye becoming opaque and the retinas becoming less sensitive. Wraparound styles will protect your eyes against light coming in from the sides.

999 Don't be afraid of cataract surgery.

Cataract surgery can give you the best vision you've had in decades! It's usually done in a hospital surgical suite—not an operating room—and you'll be home in several hours. I had cataract surgery on both eyes three years ago, and it was the first time in 60 years that I could see when I woke up in the morning, without having to grope for my glasses immediately. If your doctor tells you that you need cataract surgery, go for it!

1000 Boost the type with your browser.

Is the type on your computer screen too small for you to read comfortably? Increase the text size with your browser setting. Every web browser has a "Zoom" selection under "Settings" or "View." Click to zoom in. Or you can do it from your keyboard. On a PC, hold the Control key and click +. On a Mac, it's the Command key and +.

1001 Change the cursor arrow, too.

Maybe that little black arrow is too small to see easily. Change it to something larger, more brightly colored—maybe even a cartoon character. The Internet offers lots of free choices. YouTube offers very helpful tutorials on how to do this for both Mac and PC computers.

1002 Get better night-driving vision.

Drivers who have diabetes often report difficulty with night vision.

The reason: Darkness makes your pupils dilate more, and the more peripheral light that enters your eyes, the more nearsighted you become.

For a quick and simple solution, turn on the map light in your car for a few seconds and drive more slowly. The extra (nondirect) illumination will make your pupils contract a bit. Then wait a few seconds to see how your eyes are focusing. The result is slightly better vision and depth perception. But remember: This is a situational Band-Aid, not a fix. Go to your eye doctor for a checkup if the problem persists for three days. You may need eyeglasses just for night driving.

1003 Turn down the nighttime glare.

The pain and danger of nighttime glare can be minimized by a trip to the drugstore. Dry eyes are more hurt by—and less effective in—glare. In fact, the drier your eyes, the worse the problem. So sterile eyedrops, or blinking, or thinking about the end of the film *Lad: A Dog* (and the ensuing tears) can alleviate the situation by moistening your eyeballs. Contact lens wearers, especially, should always carry and use eyedrops!

1004 Night-lights may prevent retinopathy.

In "Photoreceptors in Diabetic Retinopathy" by Timothy S. Kern and Bruce A. Berkowitz, published in the January 7, 2015, issue of the *Journal of Diabetes Investigation*, the authors reported that darkness causes hypoxia (oxygen deprivation) in the retinas of patients with type 2 diabetes. The authors believe that the hypoxia may spur the tissue changes that occur in diabetic retinopathy. Light filtering through closed eyelids seems to prevent this oxygen starvation, so it may be wise to sleep with the light on. How much light will depend on how soundly you sleep and the condition of your retinas.

Note: While more research is needed, keeping the light near your bed on all night seems a very small, safe price to pay for preventing or delaying diabetic retinopathy.

However, it is a balance. Sleep researcher Meir H. Kryger, author of *A Woman's Guide to Sleep Disorders*, says that people sleep better in the dark. Excess light inhibits melatonin production…but melatonin makes you sleepier and helps regulate the sleep/wake cycle.

1005 Keep your edge.

Impaired vision can cause major accidents when you are using sharp tools or kitchen knives. To avoid bloodshed—yours—take an extra moment to ask yourself, "Where is my other hand? Where are all my fingers?" You may want to use protective gloves or disposable "first aid"/"examination" gloves.

1006 Adopt the Sherlock strategy.

Keep at least one magnifying glass handy. Magnifying glasses come in a variety of strengths. Some combine two magnifications—like 2X and 5X in a single lens; some include battery-operated lights. Many have cords so that you can wear them around your neck and leave your hands free. Magnifying glasses are a very inexpensive low-tech solution to many impaired-vision problems.

1007 Eye to eye.

Look in a mirror, covering one eye, then the other. If you notice blurring or missing parts, call your ophthalmologist for an early appointment. When you look in the mirror with *both* eyes, your brain mixes the images from both eyes and hides potential problems.

1008 Don't ignore those mysterious black-and-blue marks.

You start to get dressed in the morning or undressed at night—and there's a black-and-blue mark on your body that you absolutely can't recall. These little mysteries shouldn't be ignored. Bumping into furniture can be the first symptom of impaired vision.

You can use your smart phone camera to document your bruises.

1009 Deal with diminished vision.

I "lost" a black television remote on a Black Watch plaid-sheeted bed for two days, which jacked up my stress level and my blood glucose. When I found it, I stuck strips of neon yellow adhesive tape to the remote. Now I can find it immediately!

1010 Gaze deeply into your eyes.

Does a full moon make you want to gaze deeply into a pair of eyes? Great—make that shiny orb your monthly reminder to spend an extra few minutes checking the reflections that indicate your cholesterol levels.

In front of a mirror, in good light, look at the skin around your eyes and eyelids. High blood-cholesterol levels often create visible signs, like fatty growth on the lids or around the eyes. Also, check around the irises of your eyes: Are there new gray fatty deposits around each iris?

Of course, this is no substitute for having your doctor do blood-chemistry tests, but it's one more way for you to assist in monitoring your own health.

1011 Make your eye doctor your second-best friend.

No more just getting glasses from an optician, or having the discount-superstore eye doc give you a prescription after you read the eye chart. People with diabetes are susceptible to several specific diabetic eye diseases, and regular checkups by a qualified specialist can screen for problems and literally save your sight. In addition to diabetic retinopathy, a leading cause of blindness, specialists will also screen for cataracts and glaucoma, which are twice as prevalent in diabetics as in the rest of the population.

Please get a dilated-eye exam at least twice a year, especially if you've had diabetes for several years. Your insurance plan will pay for the second visit if your doctor says it's necessary.

1012 Your eyes aren't only *your* problem.

The National Eye Institute estimates that as many as 45% of all diagnosed diabetics have some degree of diabetic retinopathy. As many as 7.6 million

Americans will suffer from the disease in 2020, with an estimated 30,000 people a year going blind from this disorder. According to the Centers for Disease Control and Prevention, diabetes is the leading cause of new cases of blindness in adults. This is a growing problem as the number of people living with diabetes increases, so does the number of people with impaired vision. The CDC also states that diabetes-related blindness costs the nation about $500 million annually. Uncle Sam wants you—to get your eyes checked!

1013 **Those funny little yellow spots are serious.**

During every eye examination, your doctor should examine your retinas for little yellow spots called "drusen." They are an early warning sign of macular degeneration, a disease that is a leading cause of blindness.

If your doctor finds these fatty spots, you must check your vision every day with a quick, simple test.

Cover one eye and look at something with straight lines, like a sheet of graph paper or the Amsler grid mentioned in Tip 997. Now cover the other eye and repeat. If any of these lines appear wavy or you see a blank spot, call your doctor and get a referral to a retina specialist *immediately*.

1014 **UFOs—unidentified *floating* objects.**

These mysterious little dots are usually harmless specks of debris floating around in diabetic patients' eyes, and they often increase as we grow older.

But a *sudden* increase in these floaters—especially with changes in your vision or floating lights in one eye—should make you see your ophthalmologist *immediately*. They are early warning signs of a detached or torn retina.

1015 **Fall-proof your home.**

Most falls are caused by poor vision. People with diabetes often don't see well, and that's why they trip and fall. To prevent falling, get rid of scatter rugs or put skidproof tape on all the corners so they'll stay put. Clothing, papers, shoes, and other objects should be moved off the floor so you won't trip over them. Secure electrical and phone cords, too. And skidproof your feet. Wear shoes and slippers that have nonslip soles; don't wear socks alone.

If the soles of your feet do not have neuropathy, it may be safe to walk around your home barefoot for greater traction.

1016 **Heighten the contrast.**

To make seeing easier, use plates and dishes with contrasting colored rims and utensils with brightly colored handles.

Paint doorways or find a creative way—like an appliqued border—to dramatize the edges. Put reflector tape on every edge you can think of, then ask a friend to double-check to see if there's anything else that needs special marking.

1017 Lighten up.

According to the Visiting Nurse Service of New York, older people need three times as much light as younger ones. Many people with diabetes also need a lot more light. You may need stronger bulbs or more lamps to increase your comfort, visibility, and sense of security.

1018 Label your drugs clearly.

Those tiny little vials with even tinier print can drive us nuts and create a serious risk if we can't read the labels.

Make a special label for each drug. Take a 3"x5" index card and print on it all the necessary details so large that you can read them very easily. Then slip the index card and the drug vial into a plastic bag. Now reading all the details and taking the right medication at the right time will be easy.

1019 If you could do only one thing for your eyes.

According to continuing analysis of the Diabetes Control and Complications Trial (DCCT) and its follow-up study, Epidemiology of Diabetes Interventions and Complications (EDIC), one factor most influences the onset and progression of diabetic retinopathy.

This crucial factor is low A1C numbers. Your focusing on getting these numbers down—and keeping them there—may prevent or delay diabetic retinopathy.

1020 More about your retinas.

Need more motivation for sticking to your regimen? How about keeping your eyesight? Retinal problems begin when high blood-glucose levels thin the blood vessels, and blood leaks out of the thinned optical vein and artery walls. Your ophthalmologist can see on your retinal scans where little dots on the back wall of your eye indicate microscopic blood leaks. That's the beginning of retinal damage—and the beginning of vision loss. If you can get a copy of the photo of your retinas, keep it in your wallet and take it out to look at it whenever you need a willpower boost.

CARDIOVASCULAR

1021 Morning cardiology appointment? Skip your breakfast coffee.

The caffeine in your breakfast coffee will jack up your blood pressure at your appointment, often to the point of your cardiologist's wanting to prescribe medication for hypertension. For example, your systolic blood pressure (the top number) after coffee might be as high as 160 to 170, while without coffee it is likely to be 120 to 130. Other aspects of your cardiology exam with and without caffeine will likely differ, too, so for the most accurate morning cardiology exam, skip your breakfast coffee.

And for the most accurate afternoon cardiology exam, skip your mid-morning and lunchtime coffee.

1022 Why does my cardiologist always want to examine my ankles?

True, your ankles are a long distance from your heart, but they can give your cardiologist lots of information if they're swollen. Often your cardiologist will press a thumb into your ankles to check whether a dent remains in your flesh. This swelling is a symptom of congestive heart failure, a disease in which your heart is unable to pump well enough to maintain blood flow to your body.

There are many causes, so your cardiologist will have to run a number of tests to make a definitive diagnosis and treatment plan.

1023 High blood sugars can lead to a buildup of plaque in blood vessels.

And it's cumulative. And dangerous! Plaque can travel and wind up anywhere—in your coronary blood vessels (heart attack), carotid arteries and veins (stroke), and many other places in your body.

Keep your blood glucose under control and you can avoid these deadly problems.

1024 Type 2 diabetes and cardiovascular disease can shorten your life.

Type 2 diabetes and cardiovascular disease can shorten your life by an average of eight years. Do you really like these statistics? Think about it!

1025 There's peripheral artery disease, too.

Peripheral artery disease (PAD) can be a problem *before* your heart and coronary blood vessels are affected because your blood has to travel farther to and from your hands and feet. That's why neuropathy in your toes and feet becomes such a problem.

1026 Avoid even "high-normal" blood pressure.

According to the famed Framingham Heart Study, which celebrates its 70ᵗʰ birthday in 2018, "high-normal" blood pressure (120-139/80-89) increases the risk of cardiovascular disease, especially among patients with diabetes.

Best bet: Check your blood pressure at least three mornings a week, as soon as you get up—at the same time, if possible—and keep a log of your results. (You can buy a good blood pressure monitor for less than $50. Veridian makes one that even stores data.) Contact your cardiologist if you see unusual results.

1027 Check your blood pressure twice a day if you can.

Sad fact: Diabetes patients are much more likely to suffer from cardiovascular disease, including strokes and heart attacks, than their nondiabetic peers. Checking your blood pressure first thing in the morning and at roughly the same time in the afternoon or before dinner, and keeping a log to bring to your cardiologist, will help both of you notice any unusual changes. (Some clever little meters have a green-yellow-red light to alert you to normal, borderline, and high blood pressure readings.)

1028 *Low* blood pressure can be dangerous, too.

While we all know the risks of high blood pressure, not enough attention is given to *low* blood pressure (lower than 90/60). The second number—the diastolic, when your heart is resting between beats—is especially important.

If your diastolic number is frequently between 40 and 50, call your cardiologist for an urgent appointment. Such a low number means that your heart has to pump harder to circulate blood through your body. Your cardiologist will set a higher target of 55 to 60 to prevent cardiovascular stress and often may change your medication.

1029 Huge black-and-blue marks reveal hemorrhaging.

One of my friends got a "bad" lidocaine injection for osteoarthritis into two trigger points in her hip. Three days later, she had a massive black-and-blue mark that extended from her waist all over her buttock and hip down to six inches below her knee. Her other doctors who saw the black-and-blue mark told her that the doctor who had given her the lidocaine injection had clearly hit some major blood vessels, which caused the major subcutaneous (under the skin) hemorrhaging.

My friend's cardiologist, who saw the bruise four weeks later, taught her that hemorrhaging can take place under the skin as well as outside the skin, and she had probably lost about a pint of blood because of the extent of the bruise. (Fortunately, two months later, my friend's bruise is almost gone.)

1030 Visible veins on one leg may be an important symptom.

Does only one leg show visible veins? It may indicate that there's a blood clot somewhere, and that can be very dangerous because it can travel all over your body, causing possible damage.

1031 Pay attention to hair loss.

Diabetic nerve damage is often felt; diabetic peripheral vascular damage often isn't.

If you're losing hair on the lower part of your legs, bring it to your cardiologist's attention quickly. Hair loss here can be a symptom of vascular disease, and curbing this complication now can prevent foot or leg amputation later.

1032 Cigarettes should be your own worst enemy.

People with diabetes need to do all they can to improve and maintain good blood circulation. Smoking destroys capillaries (your tiniest blood vessels) and damages circulation, especially in your hands and feet, which are at great risk, along with your kidneys and eyes. Quitting is the only smart move, and many medical groups and localities have programs to help. If you truly haven't been able to quit yet, then cut down as much as you can.

1033 Know your risk.

The National Institutes of Health warns that middle-aged people with type 2 diabetes have the same high risk of heart attack as people without diabetes who have already had one heart attack. Monitoring carbohydrate intake isn't usually enough to manage your blood glucose levels. It's also important to watch your saturated fat and trans fat intake because high cholesterol levels are also a complication of diabetes.

1034 Pessimism is more than an attitude.

Research has shown that pessimism can increase the number of T-suppressor cells. In addition to interfering with your immune system, these cells can raise the risk of your developing heart disease. Believing that your health problems are not controllable or treatable is a dangerous supposition: It even affects the intensity of your pursuing treatment.

1035 Heart disease is not a male problem.

Although heart disease tends to be classified and treated as a "mostly male" disease by the medical community, it is the single greatest health risk for women today—greater than stroke and all cancers combined. More American women die of heart disease each year than of the next seven causes of death combined. Heart disease actually kills more women than men, although typically it strikes women an average of 10 years later.

Make sure that you discuss reducing cardiovascular risk with your doctor. Prevention is crucial because most women who die suddenly of a heart attack had no history of cardiovascular disease, but did have at least one risk factor: High cholesterol, diabetes, hypertension, or smoking.

1036 Get the right tests.

For women, a treadmill stress test is less accurate and predictive than it is for men. For proper diagnosis and treatment, it should be combined with an echocardiogram or a nuclear-imaging test.

1037 Atrial fibrillation can be more serious in women.

Atrial fibrillation (AF), an abnormally fast and irregular heartbeat, is the most common form of cardiac arrhythmia. Although men are more likely than women to develop AF, women have twice the risk of stroke after developing it, according to the landmark Framingham Heart Study.

Atrial fibrillation doesn't always show up in EKGs because those tests are so brief—only about 10 seconds. If your symptoms persist, you may need a longer test with a portable heart monitor.

As a diabetic patient, you are already at risk for atrial fibrillation and other arrhythmias. Quitting smoking is the smartest move you can make to reduce your risk because *smoking triples the risk of arrhythmias*.

1038 Learn the gender differences in symptoms of heart attack and stroke.

You probably know the traditional symptoms of heart attack and stroke in men; they've been dramatized often enough. The most common male symptom of heart attack is a sharp, clutching pain in the chest that often radiates down the arm. The most common male symptoms of stroke are a sudden weakness, numbness, or lack of coordination on one side of the body, or sudden inability to speak.

In women, the signs are much more subtle and diffuse, which makes diagnosis and immediate treatment much more difficult. Heart attack symptoms include unexplained headaches, nausea, breathlessness, and palpitation. Stroke symptoms include pain, headache, changes in consciousness, and disorientation. Perhaps Nieca Goldberg, MD, medical director, of the Joan H. Tisch Center for Women's Health at NYU Langone Medical Center, summed it up best in the title of her book: *Women Are Not Small Men.*

NEUROPATHY

1039 Qualitative sensory testing: Big name, little tests.

Don't be alarmed if your doctor recommends "qualitative sensory testing." It sounds imposing, but it's actually the use of pressure, vibration, temperature, and other stimuli on your feet and legs to check for possible nerve damage. QST is used to identify and quantify sensation loss and excessive nerve irritability. The test can help your doctor plan specific treatment.

1040 Weak Legs? Check for proximal neuropathy.

This is not the same as diabetic neuropathy of the feet, which is covered in the "Feet" section beginning on page 273.

People with type 2 diabetes and older people may experience weakness in their legs or difficulty standing after they've been sitting for a long time. The cause may be proximal neuropathy: Nerve damage also known as "femoral neuropathy" or "lumbosacral plexus neuropathy." The condition starts with pain in either of the thighs, hips, buttocks, or legs, usually on one side of the body. It's worth bringing to your doctor's attention; treatment for the weakness or pain—usually physical therapy—is typically needed.

1041 If you're the only one sweating, it's not just the heat.

Diabetic nerve damage can affect the nerves that control sweating. When autonomic neuropathy keeps your sweat glands from functioning properly, your body loses the ability to regulate your temperature, like a broken thermostat. Nerve damage can also cause profuse perspiring at night, or while you're eating. Women of a certain age who have diabetes should bring unusual sweating problems to their doctor's attention—it might not be hot flashes. Ask your diabetes doctor or neurologist about treatment for this type of nerve damage.

JOINTS AND MUSCLES

1042 Muscle cramps can mean more than exertion.

If you're getting leg or other muscle cramps, give a thought to the possible causes. Your cramps could be the result of overexertion, but they can also signal dehydration or electrolyte imbalances. If clenched leg muscles recur without obvious triggers, check with your physician.

1043 Electromyography: The test that sounds worse than it is.

People with diabetes can experience decreased muscle responses, and doctors may want to test how well your muscles respond to the electrical signals transmitted by nearby nerves. The idea of running electrical pulses into your muscles sounds scary, but it's neither as fearsome nor as painful as it sounds. Electromyography (EMG) displays your muscles' electrical activity on a screen and isolates the slower or weaker responses that suggest nerve damage. This test can also be done at the same time as nerve-conduction studies and, for most people, is not especially irritating or painful.

1044 The Psi factor.

This psi has nothing to do with ESP. It stands for pounds per square inch, a measurement of stress used by mechanical engineers and architects.

Here's why it applies to you. If you are seriously overweight, you are putting your knees and ankles at very great risk, damaging them with every step you take. There is a simple mathematical formula to estimate the pounds per square inch pressure on your knees and ankles. It is only an estimate because it ignores your height, and the taller you are, the more stress you put on your knees and ankles. However, it also underestimates the psi impact because the formula treats the entire area of the joint as if it were all bone—not flesh and bone—and your bone really bears your weight.

The formula for calculating the pounds-per-square-inch on each joint is simple…

Measure around your knee with a tape measure. This is its circumference.
Divide by 3.14 (pi) to get your knee's diameter.
Divide by 2 to get your knee's radius.
Then multiply the radius by itself and then by 3.14.

Yes, this is your old high school geometry formula for calculating the area of a circle. It really doesn't matter that your knee is shaped irregularly and is not a pure circle. The circumference controls the area; try experimenting with a string and you'll see.

To bring the damage home, let's plug in some numbers:

If your knee measures 20" in circumference, its diameter is 6.37" and its radius is 3.18". Its area is 31.7 square inches. If you weigh 150 pounds, the pressure on your knee is 4.7 psi. (A square inch is an area about the size of the first joint of your thumb.) If you weight 300 pounds, the pressure on your knee is 9.4 psi.

Your ankle's circumference is generally about 60% the size of your knee's, so the psi numbers are nearly twice as large.

Is it any wonder that seriously overweight people are at substantial risk for osteoarthritis and other joint and muscle problems?

Will knowing the potential damage persuade you to lose some weight? I certainly hope so!

1045 Step up.

Does one knee hurt more than the other?

This trick may lessen your pain: When you step up on a curb or climb steps, lead off with your "good" leg. When you step down from the curb or go downstairs, start with your "bad" leg.

1046 Dealing with frozen shoulder.

"Frozen shoulder" covers all causes of motion loss in the shoulder joint. Like many joint problems, it affects women more than men, approximately 10% to 20% of people with diabetes, and usually begins between the ages of 40 and 65. According to the American Academy of Orthopaedic Surgeons, frozen shoulder is probably caused by underlying inflammation that makes the capsule surrounding the shoulder joint thicken and contract, so that the upper arm bone (humerus) has less room to move around freely.

Nonsurgical treatment, which should be tried first, includes anti-inflammatory drugs and muscle relaxants, heat or ice therapies, physical therapy combined with stretching exercises done at home to restore motion and function, and corticosteroid injections.

Arthroscopic surgery is used if there is no improvement after several months. It must be followed by an exercise program to restore function and range of motion.

1047 Tandem Point^SM therapy may help.

Tandem Point^SM therapy can relieve pain and/or loss of motion that may be caused by muscle contraction. This form of physical therapy is a combination of acupressure and massage that involves applying pressure simultaneously to a trigger point and one or more other points, then stretching through the trigger point.

Tandem Point^{SM} therapy is fast; according to a presentation made at the National Institutes of Health, improvement is usually seen after only one visit.

1048 Lidocaine injections into trigger points may ease pain.

Trigger points are identifiable, irritable points in skeletal muscles or their covering not caused by trauma or inflammation. These painful points can feel like a little knot or band of muscle.

Lidocaine injections into trigger points are used frequently to numb the trigger points and relieve pain. They are often as effective as steroid injections, but will raise your blood glucose less. However, test your blood glucose frequently after your lidocaine injection and increase your insulin dosage, if necessary.

1049 Know the signs of diabetic muscle infarction.

Limb infarction is an area of tissue death in an arm or leg. It affects nerves and muscles when damage starts to happen after four to six hours of interference with—or stopping of—blood supply. While skeletal muscles are relatively resistant to infarction compared with the brain and heart, the major cause is long-standing, poorly controlled diabetes.

Early symptoms include coldness in an arm, hand, or leg, pain or muscle spasm in that area, numbness or tingling, or muscle weakness.

Note: These symptoms affect only one side of your body. Call EMS immediately. Also, swear to yourself that you will take better control of your diabetes. Treatment depends on the location and extent of the nerve and muscle damage.

1050 Watch for diabetic amyotrophy (proximal diabetic neuropathy).

While diabetic amyotrophy is a form of diabetic neuropathy, I've placed this tip here because this is a disease of muscle atrophy (wasting). It occurs most frequently in poorly controlled type 2 diabetic patients and affects buttock, hip, thigh, or leg muscles, usually on one side of the body, but it can spread to both sides.

Well-controlled blood glucose is the best way to prevent diabetic amyotrophy and, fortunately, the disease can be reversed through better blood-glucose control, diet, exercise, and physical therapy, which is extremely helpful.

1051 Repetitive-stress injuries don't heal very well.

As diabetes patients, we heal more slowly, and repetitive-stress injuries, which are cumulative, pile unhealed injury on top of unhealed injury. Carpal tunnel syndrome is a well-known type of this injury, although in 1700 Italian physician Bernardo Ramazzini first documented repetitive-stress injuries in more than 20 types of workers, including musicians and clerks.

When diagnosed early, repetitive-stress injuries can often be alleviated through analgesics, biofeedback, heat, physical therapy, occupational therapy, and ultrasound. Surgery should be thought of only as a last resort because diabetic patients are generally poor surgery risks.

1052 Cherries can alleviate osteoarthritis and gout pain.

Tart cherries—especially Montmorency cherries as fresh fruit, dried, or juice—protected patients with existing gout from recurrent attacks, according to a Boston University Medical Center study published in December 2012 in *Arthritis & Rheumatology*.

Cherries may also help reduce the symptoms of osteoarthritis. In a 2013 article in *Osteoarthritis and Cartilage*, researchers at Philadelphia VA Medical Center reported that patients who drank 16 ounces of tart cherry juice a day for six weeks experienced a "significant improvement in pain, stiffness and physical function."

GASTROINTESTINAL TRACT

1053 Don't be embarrassed to tell your doctor.

Galloping diarrhea, weird abdominal noises, other strange symptoms—your doctor has seen and heard it all before. Get your problems out in the open; neglecting them might cause serious problems in the future.

1054 Abdominal pains I: Is it pancreatitis?

Pancreatitis—inflammation of the pancreas—can be either acute or chronic. Eighty percent of pancreatitis cases are caused by alcohol abuse or gallstones. Gallstones are the single most common cause of acute pancreatitis, while alcohol abuse is the single most common cause of chronic pancreatitis. Type 2 diabetes is linked to a 2.8-fold higher risk of pancreatitis, according to a May 2009 study published in *Diabetes Care*. Smoking increased the risk of both acute and chronic pancreatitis.

The most common symptoms of pancreatitis are severe upper-abdominal burning pain radiating to the back, nausea, and vomiting that gets worse with eating.

Call 911 and get to an emergency room immediately if you have these symptoms.

1055 Abdominal pains II: Is it diabetic ketoacidosis?

Symptoms of diabetic ketoacidosis (DKA) usually evolve over 24 hours. DKA is a dangerous condition characterized by high blood glucose and high excretion of ketone bodies. The most common symptoms are abdominal pain that may be severe, nausea and vomiting, excessive urination and thirst, and dehydration. High blood-glucose readings are common.

A "fruity" or "acetone" breath can aid in the diagnosis.

Ketone test strips can tell patients whether they are at immediate risk for DKA, which can be toxic. In the January 2014 issue of *Diabetes Forecast*, the article "Ketone Test Strips 2014" by Erika Gebel Berg, PhD tells patients how to analyze these urine test strips for ketones.

Call 911 and get to an emergency room immediately if you suspect DKA.

1056 To outwit gastroparesis, try spacing your meals.

Neuropathy from extended high blood-glucose levels can lead to diabetic gastroparesis, taking its toll on stomach nerves and causing slow digestion, nausea, indigestion, belching, and vomiting. Doctors suggest battling the milder symptoms of stomach-nerve damage by eating small, frequent meals, avoiding fats, and eating less fiber. For more severe symptoms, doctors may prescribe erythromycin to speed digestion, metoclopramide to speed digestion and help relieve nausea, or other drugs that can affect stomach-enzyme secretions.

1057 Slow gastric emptying delays everything.

It usually takes about two hours for food and drink to move out of your stomach and into your small intestine. In slow gastric emptying, it takes at least four or five hours. Slow gastric emptying delays the absorption of drugs as well as food. Pills sit in the stomach, rather than passing through quickly. This alters the action of oral hypoglycemic medication.

Nausea and heartburn after eating are two major symptoms of slow gastric emptying. If you experience them frequently, you should probably see a gastroenterologist.

1058 A stool for your stool could help.

When "going" takes too long or is a problem, putting your feet up on a stool or bench may make it faster and easier. This discovery explains the success of entrepreneurs who are capitalizing on the marketing and selling of these devices, like Squatty Potty, but actually any piece of furniture or box that raises your feet seven to nine inches will do just fine.

1059 Balancing act.

If your blood-glucose levels run high and low and seem frequently to be 180 degrees out of sync, the problem may be that your stomach is emptying more slowly. Speak to your doctor about adjusting your insulin and possibly your oral hypoglycemic medication so that they match your digestion time better.

1060 The link between diabetes and chronic diarrhea.

Like many other systems of the body, your gastrointestinal system is affected by your diabetes. Because intestinal movement can be slowed down (gastroparesis), which is usually caused by neuropathy of the autonomic nervous system, there is a population explosion of the bacteria that normally live in the intestine, causing chronic diarrhea. Drugs that stimulate the muscular action of the intestines and antibiotics like erythromycin will usually cure chronic diarrhea.

1061 What you pass can be a clue.

Regular diarrhea or hard stools that are difficult to pass can indicate dehydration. Other signs you may be dehydrated include dark urine, infrequent urination, headaches, dry mouth, and fatigue.

KIDNEYS

1062 Watch your albumin and creatinine.

Guidelines from the National Kidney Foundation suggest that people with diabetes, hypertension, or a family history of kidney disease should get a urine test for albumin and a blood test for creatinine. Your diabetes doctor will tell you how often they are needed, which often depends on how long you have had diabetes and how well controlled your blood glucose is. The albumin test indicates impaired function (a qualitative test), and the creatinine test tells your doctor how efficiently your kidneys are functioning (a quantitative test).

1063 Know your numbers I: Albumin

Your doctor should be having your urine tested for protein regularly, as detailed in the above tip. When your kidneys are functioning normally, they filter out a protein called albumin from your urine. (Tiny amounts of albumin are called "microalbumin.") As kidney function declines, more and more albumin escapes into the urine.

Get a copy of every lab test and examine it. According to Quest Diagnostics, numbers between 0 and 30 are normal. Ask your doctor to evaluate any higher number that might be abnormal.

1064 Know your numbers II: Creatinine.

Creatinine is a white crystalline compound that is a component of urine. Results are converted to mg/liter. Not only should you look at whether the results of any one test are normal, but you and your doctor should compare them with the past two or three results to make sure that they are not sliding slowly from normal to abnormal.

1065 Know your numbers III: Glomerular filtration rate (GFR).

Simply put, the glomerular filtration rate (GFR) tells you and your doctor at what percentage your kidneys are doing their work. The National Kidney Foundation lists six stages of chronic kidney disease, based on your GFR...

STAGE	DESCRIPTION	GLOMERULAR FILTRATION RATE (GFR)
At increased risk	Risk factors for kidney disease (e.g., diabetes, high blood pressure, family history, older age, ethnic group)	More than 90
1	Kidney damage (protein in the urine) and normal GFR	More than 90
2	Kidney damage and *mild* decrease in GFR	60 to 89
3	*Moderate* decrease in GFR	30 to 59
4	*Severe* decrease in GFR	15 to 29
5	Kidney failure (dialysis or kidney transplant needed)	Less than 15

1066 Early kidney disease in type 1 diabetes may be reversible.

Microalbinuria (small amounts of protein in the urine), an early sign of kidney disease, might be reversed with early detection and good blood-glucose control. The PERL (Preventing Early Renal Loss in Diabetes) study will test whether the drug allopurinol can prevent or slow kidney disease in type 1 diabetics.

Factors that make a difference in returning to normal kidney function include early detection of microalbinuria, a hemoglobin A1C of less than 8.0, systolic blood pressure less than 115, total cholesterol less than 198, and fasting triglycerides under 145. The study will be completed in the summer of 2019.

Let's hope for good news!

FEET

1067   Check your feet morning or night.

Your feet need checking at least once a day. So mentally tie foot-checking to something else you do without fail, like brushing your teeth or locking the door. Once you've linked this task to a routine, it will take as little conscious effort to remember checking your feet as it does to brush your teeth.

Remember to check for cuts, bruises, calluses, "hot spots," and anything that wasn't there at your last inspection.

1068   Don't be de-feet-ed.

Until I interviewed a doctor with years of experience in family medicine, I was under the misunderstanding that most diabetic patients' trips to the emergency room were for hypoglycemia.

Not so. Many more visits are for foot problems, such as splinters, infections, or swelling, which often start small, but become worse very rapidly. Taking the best care of your feet will keep you out of emergency rooms and hospitals.

1069   Your odds are one in four, so start watching now.

Without vigilance and prevention, your odds of foot problems are one in four. Of the 30 million Americans with diabetes, seven million will develop foot problems related to the disease. Poor circulation can cause a lack of sensitivity and the loss of the ability to feel pain, heat, and cold. That makes it possible to develop cuts, scrapes, blisters, or pressure sores without feeling them. And if minor injuries go untreated, complications could lead to ulceration and possibly even amputation. So if you "just don't bother" to examine your feet every day, remember your one-in-four odds.

1070   Having cold feet means more than reluctance.

At the very least, cold feet are a sign of poor peripheral (your hands and feet) circulation. More seriously, cold feet might be a symptom of neuropathy, which often affects diabetic feet. Keep your feet warm with the most comfortable socks you can find—cashmere-blend knee socks go on sale the day after Christmas.

Tell your doctor about your cold feet at your next appointment.

1071   Never use an electric blanket on your feet.

If you have neuropathy, you could burn your feet with an electric blanket and not realize the damage until it's too late. You can use the electric blanket on the rest of your body, and a hot-water bottle is safe for your feet. (Or teach your cats and dogs to sleep on your feet—that's the origin of Three-Dog Night.)

1072 Custom orthotics may not be necessary.

Try the orthotics and insoles sold at your pharmacy first. In one recent visit, I found more than 20 different types, none of which cost more than $20 for the largest men's size. Definitely worth trying!

1073 Foot neuropathy? Increase your flexibility and circulation.

When your toes get stiff and inflexible, walking becomes difficult. You may even need to use a cane or a walker.

Try this little trick to increase your circulation and flexibility. Pick up marbles with your toes. Start with large marbles and graduate to small ones. You can also pick up napkin rings with your toes and put them on a spike. (A popular toy for infants and toddlers consists of concentric rings that are placed on a peg. Buy it for yourself and give your toes a challenge.)

1074 Foot ulcers are deadly.

True story: Several months ago, I ran into a neighborhood friend, and we brought each other up to date. She knows that I have diabetes—but not that I was writing this book—and told me that one of her neighbors, a woman in her forties with poorly controlled diabetes, had been found dead in her apartment several days earlier. The cause of death was an untreated foot ulcer that became infected.

Without belaboring the point, untreated foot ulcers can kill you. If you have a sore on your foot, call your doctor *immediately, or visit the nearest urgent-care facility.*

1075 "Diabetic foot" covers a lot of ground.

"Diabetic foot" sums up a cluster of serious problems common to people with diabetes: Neuropathy, vasculopathy (circulatory problems), infections, and poor wound healing.

If your doctor diagnoses your problem as "diabetic foot," ask for a more specific diagnosis and a detailed treatment plan.

1076 "Charcot foot" means only one thing.

Charcot foot is a specific disease. It begins with neuropathy and progresses quickly to a degenerative arthritis in which the ligaments and joint surfaces of the metatarsal and tarsal bones disintegrate.

According to the American Diabetes Association, 60% to 70% of people with diabetes develop peripheral neuropathy that can lead to Charcot foot, whose onset usually occurs in middle-aged patients who have had diabetes for 15 to 20 years. Of course, poorly controlled blood glucose makes the situation worse—and earlier.

Treatment can be complex and can take months. The damaged joint must be stabilized for at least two months, which means that it must not bear any weight. Patients are prescribed bed rest and/or a walking cast and crutches. If there is no improvement, surgery to correct the damaged ligaments and joints may be necessary.

1077 Socks can be your best friend.

Anything that rubs against your feet is very bad. Anything that protects and soothes them is very good. So start your collection of colorful cotton socks. The importance of the warmth, protection, and absorbency of soft cotton socks can't be overemphasized. Wear them under heavier socks in bad weather.

1078 Hurting? Your drugstore has topical help.

People with diabetes often experience pain in their feet as the nerves become damaged from continued high blood glucose levels. Some people report lying awake at night, trying to sleep despite their discomfort

Go for a topical analgesic: "Stop Pain" spray or even Anbesol—a product made for teething babies and oral cold-sore sufferers—can help. If it's safe enough to put in your mouth, it's safe enough for unbroken skin on your foot. By dulling or removing the pain temporarily, you are freed to think about something else, or even to get a good night's sleep.

1079 Diabetic socks are not a crock.

Don't make the mistake of thinking that all products pitched at people with diabetes are after your money. So-called "diabetic socks" can change your life! Some are made with wider tops because tight or binding socks can restrict your circulation, which is the last thing you want or need. Some are made with patented "miracle fibers" that wick away moisture and/or prevent rubbing and chafing. If your feet are giving you any trouble at all, check out socks designed to answer these problems. Yes, you'll pay more for them; and yes, anything that helps your feet last throughout your lifetime is worth that extra outlay.

1080 Why go barefoot when slippers were made just for you?

The selection and ingenuity behind foot-problem slippers will amaze you. The uglier term is "edema footwear," also known as "diabetic footwear," but the comfort and relief from these specialty products will surprise you when you check them out. Special shoes and slippers have been designed to help patients suffering from edema (swelling), sensitive skin, misshapen feet, and other problems. And they're not your grandmother's black old-lady shoes. Attractive and comfortable styles now exist in extra-wide, no-inside-seams, down-lined—whatever you need to prevent or relieve problems. Don't wait until foot pain sends you looking for them—wearing them preventively is doubly smart. Search "diabetic footwear" in a web browser, and you'll find many places to shop.

1081 Walk barefoot where it's safe.

You can tell a lot about diabetic neuropathy in your feet by walking barefoot in your home. Feel the difference between carpets, wooden floors, tile, or marble floors. Be especially sensitive to any numbness in your toes—that's where neuropathy starts.

1082 Ask your doctor about Plastazote.

Footwear and orthotics play a key role in foot care for people with diabetes, both to prevent and to help heal. Plastazote foam is the most often used material for protecting diabetic feet that have lost their sensitivity, and orthotics utilizing Plastazote can relieve pressure "hot spots" by conforming to heat and pressure. Because Plastazote shapes to your feet, it provides both comfort and protection. Ask your doctor about shoe inserts made with this product, or a similar one. You can buy them from many online retailers.

1083 Watch your feet in the winter.

One of the hardest things for some people to remember is that "familiar" does not equal "safe." Just because you've lived in Buffalo or Cleveland for years and are used to the weather doesn't mean your feet won't need special attention in the winter. Cold feet—especially wet, cold feet—can be disastrous for people with diabetes. Seamless socks and lined waterproof boots are vital in the winter! Check your feet often; someone without diabetic neuropathy might feel developing frostbite, but you might not. Keep your feet warm and dry. If possible, have someone else dig your car out of the snowbank or shovel your walk. And carry an extra pair of shoes and socks with you or in your car, in case yours become wet.

1084 Beach shoes are a must!

Walking barefoot in the sand really works only in films. The sand that looks so inviting from a distance is actually mined liberally with sharp-edged seashells and discarded sharp-edged cans. And it's hot! Always wear shoes at the beach or on hot pavement, and put sunscreen with a high SPF on the tops of your feet. Semirigid soled, net-topped beach shoes make you look like a savvy surfer—too smart to risk unnecessary hazards as you enjoy nature at the shore.

1085 Go with the flow.

One of the smartest, effortless things you can do for your feet is to keep the blood flow going. Put your feet up when you are sitting to increase circulation, and don't cross your legs for long periods. No tight socks unless you're wearing compression socks for edema, and no elastic or garters on your legs. And if you've been sitting awhile, wiggle your toes and rotate your ankles to improve blood flow in your feet and legs.

1086 The right way to treat your feet.

Soothing emollients on your feet are always welcomed, but rub skin lotion or cream *only* on the tops and bottoms of your feet. *Never* put lotion between your toes; the warm, moist climate there could invite athlete's foot and other nasties. And note any changes on your feet that last too long.

How long is too long? Call your doctor immediately if a cut, sore, blister, or bruise on your foot does not clearly begin to heal after one day.

1087 Break in new shoes slowly.

Never wear new shoes all day away from home; this includes new sneakers. Carry a spare pair with you just in case. Break in new shoes first at home. If they are uncomfortable, return them. (Most stores and online retailers will let you return them within 30 days even if you've worn them outside your house.) You do not want to risk getting a blister because blisters can become infected and turn dangerous in a matter of hours.

1088 Anodyne therapy: Worth checking out.

If foot ulcers or damaged nerves in your legs and feet give you grief, consider anodyne therapy. In this treatment, infrared light-emitting "paddles" are placed over damaged areas to reduce pain by improving your circulation. You'll need 12 to 24 sessions of 30 to 40 minutes each, according to podiatrists, but results are reported to last for one year, with about 90% of patients obtaining relief. For more information, call Anodyne Therapy, LLC, (800) 521-6664, or log on to AnodyneTherapy.com.

1089 Casting call.

Untreated foot sores or ulcers may lead to amputation. Previously, these problems were treated with special shoes, but many patients did not comply with their doctors' orders and took off the shoes.

To solve this problem, researchers at the Pitié Salpêtrière teaching hospital in Paris invented a virtually unremovable fiberglass cast that helps diabetic foot sores heal faster than the shoes did. That's probably because only one determined patient in the study was able to remove the cast, compared with many who simply stopped wearing the shoes. This fiberglass cast is now being used in the United States; ask your diabetes doctor if they would help you and, if so, to prescribe them.

1090 Keep your feet dry when gardening.

Heavy watering means taking special care of your feet. Apply petroleum jelly or a urea-based lotion on the bottoms of your feet, and then cover with cotton socks and rubber boots. Not only will your feet feel completely dry, but they will think they're getting a spa treatment.

1091 Have your favorite shoes stopped fitting?

If your favorite shoes have stopped being comfy, it may be an early sign of foot trouble. Double-check by trying on several pairs of your favorites, especially at the beginning of spring and fall. Tightness can indicate swelling or "hot spots"—blisters waiting to happen. Tell your doctor, and you may want to buy new shoes. Depending on where you live, you may want different shoes for warm and cold seasons.

1092 Keep soaking time short.

You'd think that soaking your feet for a while would alleviate dryness problems, but prolonged soaking actually causes dryness. Limit soaking your feet to 10 minutes at a time, and dry them carefully—especially between your toes. Keep your showers short, too.

1093 Baby your feet with powder.

In order to prevent dampness between your toes, which can cause fungus to develop, keep the skin between your toes dry by using cotton swabs or powder. Baby powder has a pleasant unisex aroma, but many people find lavender more appealing, and women may prefer rose-scented powder.

1094 Nail it down.

Thick or yellow toenails can be a symptom of two different diseases: One caused by a fungus, one by bacteria. Call your doctor as soon as you notice this problem. Like many others, treatment is easier and faster if the problem is caught early.

1095 Mirror, mirror.

If you can't see your feet to examine them—tops and soles—use a mirror on a stand and a magnifying glass in a well-lighted area.

1096 Leave corns and calluses to your doctor.

Having diabetes means that you shouldn't practice self-taught surgery on your feet. Do not cut corns or calluses; broken skin can lead to infection. However, you can use a pumice stone to smooth them. Rub gently in *one direction only* to avoid tearing the skin. If you tear or cut your skin accidentally, apply triple-antibiotic cream to the injury and cover with an adhesive bandage. Change the bandage every day. If it does not begin to heal within three days, call your doctor or visit an urgent-care center.

1097 Pedicure pointers.

Spring and summer, a cruise, or a sunny resort are all invitations to show off our pretty feet. And that means a pedicure.

To prevent damage, you'll have to lay down the law to make sure the pedicurist doesn't do anything that could cause an infection. That means no cutting or shaving of cuticles or corns, but cutting toenails carefully is safe. Emery boards and pumice stones are even safer.

1098 Shoe smarts.

Buy shoes that are long enough, wide enough, and deep enough so that they don't pinch, rub, or squeeze your feet. All of these irritations can cause blisters. Shop for shoes at the end of the day, when your feet are at their largest. And try them on with the socks, stockings, or tights you plan to wear with them. You'll be able to gauge whether they fit properly, and you'll get a better idea of how they'll look together.

1099 Step lively!

There you are, bopping along happily in an even rhythm. This is a good time to pay attention to your feet. Are there any numb spots? Any painful ones? Take notes and call your podiatrist.

1100 The synergy of socks.

If your feet ache from cold or neuropathy, try putting on a second pair of soft, cushiony, nonbinding socks on top of the first pair. For reasons understood by physicians, physicists, physiologists, and leprechauns, the effect is more than twice as soothing and warming as a single pair. Try it!

1101 Lengthening your Achilles tendon may prevent recurrent foot ulcers.

Diabetic foot ulcers can be healed and their recurrence can be prevented, according to the findings of a two-year study at the Washington University School of Medicine in St. Louis, which were published in the August 2003 issue of *Journal of Bone and Joint Surgery*. All the participants received total-contact casts; half of them also had their Achilles tendons lengthened, outpatient surgery that generally takes only 15 minutes. Two years after treatment, foot ulcers had recurred in 81% of the cast-only group, but in only 38% of the subjects who had undergone the Achilles tendon surgery.

HANDS

1102 Easier kitchen tools.

Little things can make a big difference in your quality of life. Gadgets that are easier to manipulate can diminish the pain in your hands and fingers considerably. Some of the most useful I've found are a ridged rubber mat about the size of a pot holder that makes it easier to open screw-top jars and a can opener with ergonomic handles.

1103 Non-child-resistant prescription bottles minimize hand pain.

Child-resistant prescription bottles are hard to open, especially if you have arthritis or other hand problems. If you don't have small children, get your prescriptions in easy-to-open pop-top containers.

1104 Gloves aren't for wimps.

Gloves protect your hands from chapping and dryness caused by cold and windburn. People with diabetes need to be especially protective of their hands to prevent skin damage and even possible frostbite. Try wearing knitted silk gloves under your winter gloves—they're available through outdoor and ski shops and catalogs—or wear two pairs of gloves at one time.

1105 American hot wax.

A paraffin treatment for your hands can reduce arthritis pain and increase the flexibility of your hands and fingers. No need to visit a nail spa, unless you want to try a treatment first. You should be able to buy the whole kit to treat both hands and feet for under $75. You can reuse the paraffin and use the treatment several times a week.

Note: These kits often go on sale right after Christmas.

1106 Carpal tunnel syndrome I: Know the symptoms.

Your fingers may feel numb, or like pins and needles. If these strange feelings persist for more than a day—and especially if you spend a good part of the day at the computer or doing repetitive actions with your hands—carpal tunnel syndrome is a likely diagnosis.

1107 Carpal tunnel syndrome II: It's all in the wrist.

Carpal tunnel syndrome is caused by repeated physical stress to a small part of the wrist, which then squeezes a major nerve. High blood glucose may also damage collagen in your wrist, which can also increase pressure on this nerve.

1108 Carpal tunnel syndrome III: Splint, steroids, surgery.

The most conservative and sensible treatment starts with your doctor splinting your wrist to keep it stabilized and free of pressure. You'll have to wear the splint as much as possible—even at night.

The next step is steroid injections to reduce the swelling putting pressure on the nerve. (Blood glucose levels can shoot up for three or four days after steroid injections, so you'll have to increase your diabetes medications.)

Surgery may be necessary if your pain becomes severe, or if your hand and wrist muscles start to weaken noticeably.

1109 Trigger finger, trigger thumb.

They sound like fightin' words from a John Wayne western, but they're a common problem for people with diabetes who are over the age of 40.

Trigger finger and trigger thumb occur when the finger's flexor tendon or sheath thickens or swells, preventing normal, smooth gliding. When this tendon swells too much, it gets stuck and locks or clicks. Very often age causes this swelling, and it can be prevented by frequently massaging your fingers.

Your doctor can diagnose trigger finger and trigger thumb by examining your fingers and manipulating them, checking if there is a catching or locking as they move. X rays are not necessary.

Treatment is similar to that for carpal tunnel syndrome: Splinting, sometimes taking aspirin, ibuprofen, or another anti-inflammatory drug to reduce the swelling, and a steroid injection or surgery if necessary.

1110 The easiest way to get a blood sample for blood-glucose testing.

Because of anatomy and physiology, it's easier to get a blood sample from the outside of your finger (pinky side) than the inside (thumb side).

Best fingers to use: Ring and middle finger. Avoid your pointer finger—it has too many nerves.

TEETH

1111 Six-month checkups are especially important.

People with diabetes are at higher risk for tooth decay, periodontal (gum) disease, fungal infections of the mouth, and oral infection and delayed healing. Six-month—or even more frequent—visits to your dentist can prevent these problems, or stop them in their earliest stages. Think of the difference between having a cavity filled and needing to have that tooth extracted and replaced!

1112 Get screened for oral cancer.

Make sure that your dentist examines your mouth for oral cancer once a year. Oral cancer is more prevalent in African-Americans, men, people over the age of 45, and people who use alcohol and tobacco, including smokeless types. However, there is no statistical correlation between people with diabetes and oral cancer.

Your dentist should examine the floor of your mouth, the front and sides of your tongue, and your soft palate to do a complete screening.

1113 More frequent cleaning saves big bucks.

Getting your teeth cleaned three or four times a year rather than twice can be a smart move. People with diabetes are more likely to develop plaque and tartar, which can lead to gingivitis and periodontal disease. More frequent professional cleaning will get rid of the plaque and tartar before they cause damage.

1114 This thrush is no bird.

If your blood-glucose levels are consistently too high, you may develop thrush, a fungal disease of the mouth characterized by white patches.

Thrush is not very serious, but it needs to be treated with oral antifungal medication, and it can raise your blood glucose substantially until it is cured.

If you develop thrush every few months, regard it as a sign that your immune system may need help. Keeping tighter control of your blood glucose is a key step.

1115 Attack your plaque.

Plaque is the sticky film on teeth that is produced by and encourages the growth of bacteria in your mouth. It is the first stage of periodontal disease and leads to the formation of calculus (calcified plaque), which builds up under the gums, forming pockets of infection.

Get rid of plaque by brushing and flossing at least twice a day, and you can avoid this nasty, expensive progression.

1116 The sugar in your saliva.

You knew this was the culprit, didn't you? People with good glycemic control have no more periodontal disease than nondiabetics. But many types of bacteria thrive on sugars, and a warm, dark, high-sugar environment—like your mouth—is ideal for growing the germs that cause gum disease.

The better your blood glucose control, the more you will protect your mouth from periodontal disease.

1117 Antibiotics reduce risk after oral surgery.

People with diabetes are at risk of infection anytime their skin is cut, and that includes oral surgery—especially because the human mouth is always teeming with bacteria. Ask your periodontist whether you should have antibiotics if the pockets of your gums will be cleaned, or if you will have root planing.

Make it a habit to ask your dentist for antibiotics whenever you have even the most minor dental work. They can prevent major problems from arising.

SKIN

1118 Save your skin.

One of the side effects of diabetes is aged-looking skin as connective tissue breaks down. One home remedy to help you hold the line—or hold off the lines!—is jojoba butter mixed with the herb gotu kola. The University of Michigan Medical School Health Library lists gotu kola as beneficially affecting collagen to inhibit scar tissue, and thus is often used to treat burn victims. A trip to the health-food store for standardized extract of gotu kola containing 40% asiaticosides (the active ingredient) and jojoba butter will make your skin look better.

1119   Minimize damage from insect bites.

The summer of 2016 brought a plague of biting insects to a large part of the United States, some of them mosquitoes, carrying the dangerous Zika virus. Many people with diabetes who hadn't been bitten in many years suddenly became human pincushions and blood banks. It's probably our sweeter blood that makes us such appealing targets!

Every one of these bites can become infected, and that's the problem for us diabetics. Prevent infection by washing the bites immediately with soap and water, putting triple antibiotic cream (bacitracin+neomycin+polymyxin B) on them, and then covering them with small adhesive bandages. And use insect repellent to prevent those bites!

1120   Recognize minor skin problems.

Except for "diabetic foot" (see page 273), most diabetic skin problems are minor, according to a New York dermatologist with over 30 years of experience. They deserve discussion because your knowing what they are and that they are not serious should alleviate your stress. Learn to recognize them and point them out to your doctor, but don't worry about them unless you notice a change in their appearance.

1121   Minor skin problems I: Dermopathy.

"Dermopathy" means "skin disease." Diabetic dermopathy occurs mostly on the shins, where some areas scar and develop dark pigment (hyperpigmentation). Other areas can atrophy (shrivel) slightly. Diabetic dermopathy can be linked to poorly controlled diabetes, but also to minor injuries and to aging. It is more of a cosmetics issue and doesn't require treatment. The dark pigment areas can be covered by makeup if they bother you.

1122   Minor skin problems II: Diabetic bullae.

Diabetic bullae are blisters on the feet and legs caused by impaired healing resulting from poor blood-glucose control. Dermatologists see them frequently and treat them with antibiotics. Tighter blood-glucose control is the best prevention and treatment.

1123   Minor skin problems III: Digital sclerosis.

Digital sclerosis is a thickening of the skin of the toes, fingers, and hands. There may be callusing and less sensitivity. About one-third of patients with type 1 diabetes have digital sclerosis, but it can be improved by getting blood glucose under control. No definitive treatment exists, but researchers are working on the problem.

1124 Minor skin problems IV: Scleroderma.

Literally "hard skin," scleroderma is an abnormal thickening of the skin of the nape of the neck and upper back, making the area feel hard to the touch. It is caused by an overproduction of collagen and is treated symptomatically by applying prescription and nonprescription lotions and creams for dry skin. Tighter blood-glucose control may help.

1125 Minor skin problems V: Carotenia.

Carotenia is a yellowing of the skin, especially of the face, palms, and soles of the feet. It occurs mostly in fair-skinned patients.

In food faddists, carotenia is caused by eating enormous quantities of fruits or vegetables containing carotene, a red- or orange-pigmented phytochemical that is converted to vitamin A. But in people with diabetes, the cause is still a mystery.

Carotenia is harmless. It is not a sign of jaundice.

1126 Minor skin problems VI: Acanthosis nigricans.

Acanthosis nigricans is the medical term that describes "velvety" thick (hyperkeratosis), abnormally increased coloration (hyperpigmentation), warty overgrowths in areas of the body where there are skin folds—especially the neck, the groin, and the underarms. This condition is related to obesity. In most cases, the condition is benign, but should be checked at every doctor's appointment to make sure there have been no changes in these growths. Treatment consists of losing weight and taking drugs that make insulin more powerful.

1127 Minor skin problems VII: Necrobiosis lipoidica.

Necrobiosis lipoidica (NL) is a skin disease characterized by collagen degeneration, thickening of blood-vessel walls, and the deposit of fat. While rare, NL occurs mostly in poorly controlled diabetics and is more common in women. Treatment consists of support stockings, elevation of the legs, and sometimes the application of topical steroids, such as psoralen, a drug used for psoriasis, followed by UVA (ultraviolet A) therapy.

1128 Minor skin problems VIII: Those nasty paper cuts.

People with diabetes frequently have thin, dry skin and less than 20/20 vision, a perfect setup for paper cuts. Delayed healing means that these little cuts are susceptible to further injury and infection.

Prevent paper cuts by regularly applying moisturizer to your hands and consider wearing examination gloves to protect your hands if you are dealing with a lot of papers.

If you don't want to see the doctor for a little paper cut, wash the area carefully and apply nonprescription triple antibiotic (bacitracin+neomycin+polymyxin B) cream. Cover it with an adhesive bandage. Or ask your doctor for a prescription for Cleocin, a liquid antibiotic that penetrates the skin better than the antibiotic cream.

1129 Minor skin problems IX: Impaired healing.

Your doctor knows how "really delayed" the healing of your skin is. Most doctors urge their patients to contact them if there is no sign of healing in two days, or if their blood-glucose numbers skyrocket. Appropriate treatment depends on the type of skin injury or problem, its location, and its extent. Seriously delayed healing may call for stitches or even surgery.

LADIES AND GENTLEMEN

1130 Make mine menopause.

Women's hormonal cycles affect their blood-glucose levels, and menopause does, too. Menopause is defined as the point when women have not had a menstrual period for 12 consecutive months. If you have diabetes, you can expect to start menopause a bit sooner—but that could be anywhere between 40 and 70! A good indicator of the age when you might reach this phase of your life is your mother's age when she reached menopause. The transition period when menstruation is erratic can last eight to 10 years before menstruation stops altogether.

1131 Mammograms are mandatory.

Premenopausal women with long-standing type 1 diabetes are particularly susceptible to a rare condition called "diabetic mastopathy," fibrous masses in the breast. The cause isn't fully understood, but doctors do know that women with diabetic mastopathy develop single or multiple firm or hard breast lumps that are not tender to the touch and that move easily under the skin. In order to reassure yourself that these recurring lumps are not malignant, women with diabetes should get mammograms, ultrasound, and even fine-needle aspirations when prescribed to keep track of these lumps and to spare themselves unnecessary surgical procedures—and worries.

1132 **Gentlemen, can we talk?**

One of the least appealing aspects of diabetes in men is the problem of impaired blood flow to private parts, and the possible resulting impotence. See a urologist as soon as possible.

Best bet: Find one who has many patients with diabetes. If you lose weight, it WILL improve your sex life!

1133 **Find help for a touchy issue.**

The internet offers many medically respected articles about diabetes in men. Here are a few to start off…

•**American Diabetes Association:** Diabetes.org/living-with-diabetes/treatment-and-care/men/

•**Joslin Diabetes Center:** Joslin.org/info/diabetes_and_sexual_health_in_men_understanding_the_connection.html

•**National Institute of Diabetes and Digestive and Kidney Diseases:** NIDDK.nih.gov/health-information/diabetes/overview/preventing-problems/sexual-urologic-problems

1134 **Don't limit yourself to narrowly defined sex.**

Physical contact is a basic human need, and needn't be limited to just the "working parts" you used in your youth. Very satisfying sex lives are possible for people whose diabetes has caused circulatory problems that affect erections or vaginal response. Rather than focusing on what's not working as you'd hoped, add empathy and foreplay and love and sharing to your experience. Remember, there's more than one way to achieve orgasm.

1135 **What if it's not bad, it's just different?**

Ladies, if your man has diabetes, circulatory or nerve damage may necessitate patience and understanding that you haven't had to use before. Don't be critical or afraid of any delays or premature ejaculation. If he's suddenly reluctant, initiate, especially if that changes the pattern of interaction between you. As he's got changes going on, your new creativity may be most welcome. Don't worry if he seems satisfied but doesn't ejaculate; he could be free to enjoy caresses and the sensual pleasures of extended foreplay—if he can get past any self-judgments or comparisons to real or imagined past prowess.

1136 **Your partner's sexual response isn't a judgment on you.**

Please be clear about one thing: Any inability of your partner to achieve a firm erection or lots of vaginal lubrication is not a judgment of your attractiveness or the state of your relationship. A man's erectile ability is physiologically dependent on blood flow and nerve response; a woman's capacity to lubricate may also be affected by neuropathy. One of the best boosts you can offer yourself and your partner is to remember that it's not about your adequacy to provide inspiration, it's about two people caring for each other's feelings and needs.

1137   **You and your diabetes are a work in progress.**

This isn't Pollyanna talking. Many improvements in diabetes care are on the horizon and should be available in the next five or 10 years. (Just remember diabetes drugs 10 years ago and you'll know what I mean.) Me? I'm looking forward to the next new drugs. How about mental insulin, which will let you just THINK your dosage? Why not dream big?

    You will make the greatest difference in what happens with your diabetes. It only gets better from here!

Acknowledgments

This book owes so much to the help of many people, for whose time, interest, and enthusiasm I am much indebted.

Special thanks to Margot Cooperman, Nao Esons, the late Gail W. Hoffmann, RN, Zvi Jankelowitz, Mary Ann Liberatore, Michael L. McQuown, Joyce Ravid, Elly Rumelt, and prolific contributor Natalie Windsor.

I am also grateful to Penny Asbell, MD, FACS, MBA, Robin N. Ginsburg, MD, Elana Maser, MD, Mary Ann McLaughlin, MD, MPH, FACC, Margaret O'Boyle, RN, Alan Schleier, DO, Gal Sivan, Aida C. Vega. MD, and especially Ronald Tamler, MD, PhD, MBA, CNSC, CDE, Clinical Director, Mount Sinai Diabetes Center.

At Bottom Line Inc., Marjory E. Abrams, my publisher and editor, is a dream to work with. Kudos also to Bottom Line Book's production team: Adrienne Makowski, John Niccolls, and Maureen Naccari.

This book would not exist without the unflagging support of Claudia Menza, my agent of many years and my friend for even longer.

Finally, my deepest thanks go to my family and friends for their constant love, patience, and enthusiastic cheerleading.

Index

Infarction
  cardiac (heart attack), 263–265
  diabetic muscle (limb), 268
Infection
  feet, 274, 277, 279
  fungal, 214, 221, 277, 279, 282–283
  hospital-acquired (HAI), 128–129
  hospital hand washing, 128
  insect bites, 284
  splinters, 121
  teeth and mouth care, 282–283
  toenails, 279
Information and questions.
  See also specific topics
  child and parent, 227–228, 231–232
  doctors, 15, 25, 103, 105, 111, 116, 127
  drugs, 15, 25
  hospital, 127–128
Internet resources, 248, 287
Injection site rotation, 21
In-network doctors, 132
Insect bites, 284
Instincts, 126, 244
Instructions
  doctor-specified personal care, 120
  drugs, 18
  hospital discharge, 130
  school care, 224
Insulin
  extra amounts, 7
  fast- vs. long-acting, 9, 21, 26–27
  flexible, 14
  half-unit dosage, 3, 8
  implantable, 29
  injection site rotation, 21
  lab-grown, 29
  premixed 70/30 vs. 75/25, 20
  replacing frequently, 12
  sick day units, 256
  storage, 12, 21
  temporary or timing, 10
  type 2 diabetes, child, 211
Insulin-dependent. *See* Type 1 diabetes
Insulin pens, 17, 26–28
Insulin pumps, 6–7, 233–234

Insulin-resistant. *See* Type 2 diabetes
Insulin weight gain, 22–23
Insurance, 22, 109–110, 114, 131–133
Insurance cards, 119
Internet pharmacies, 19
Internet resources, 248, 287
Interval training, 150
Invokana, 27
Isometric exercise, 144
Itching, 214, 221–222, 233

J
Jardiance, 27
Jell-O, 34
Joints, 266–269. *See also* Muscles
  Charcot foot, 274–275
  frozen shoulder, 267
  knees, 267
  leading with "good" leg, 267
  osteoarthritis, 62, 80, 267, 269
  overweight and, 266–267
  pounds/square inch pressure, 266–267
Jojoba butter with gotu kola, 283
Journal, 183
July, avoiding hospital and ER in, 121
Jumping, 157, 161
Jump rope, 153–154
Juvenile diabetes. *See* Type 1 diabetes, child
Juvenile Diabetes Research Foundation, 232

K
Kaffeeklatsch, 184
Kaleidoscope, 170
Kazoo, 168
Ketone test strips, 270
Kidney function, 271–272
Kitchen, 83, 136, 197, 242, 257, 280
Knees, 267
Knee-to-chest, airplane, 154
Knitting, 58
Ko-Ko song update, 193

L
Labeling, of child at school, 227, 232
Labels, food, 35, 65, 91
Labels on drug bottles, 260
Lab-grown insulin, 29

Lab tests, 105, 110, 127, 271–272
LADA (Latent Autoimmune Diabetes in Adults), 1
Lancet, 6, 18–20
Lantus insulin, 9–10, 21, 27–28
Latent Autoimmune Diabetes in Adults (LADA), 1
Laughter, 153, 165–166, 169, 183, 189–190
Legal right to choose hospital, 117–118, 123
Leg raises, 142, 144
Legs. *See also* Exercise; Walking
  ankle swelling, 261
  blisters, 284
  cardiovascular health, 261, 263
  diabetic bullae, 284
  leading with "good," 267
  muscle cramps, 266
  necrobiosis lipoidica (NL), 285
  weakness, 265
Lemons, 62, 171
Lettuce wrap, 34
Levemir insulin pen, 27
Lidocaine, 250, 268
Life curveballs, 194
Lifelong learning, 169
Lifesavers (candy), 250–252
Lifestyle adjustment, 200
Light, eyes and vision, 260
Light weights, 145–146, 159
Lipid profile test, 105
Liver profile test, 105
Living alone
  balance improvement, 245
  basement safety, 245
  bathroom, 240
  bedroom, 238, 240, 244
  blood-glucose monitoring, 242
  buddy system, 237, 239
  canes, 237–239
  celebrating privacy, 235, 240, 246
  common wall signal, 236
  contractors, 243
  emergency preparedness, 239, 242–243, 245
  falls, 243–246
  fire extinguisher, 242
  flashlight, 244–245

About the Author

Judith H. McQuown is the author of twelve books, including the best-selling *Inc. Yourself: How to Profit by Setting Up Your Own Corporation,* which has been in continuous print since 1977 and has sold over 800,000 copies. She has been an insulin-dependent type 1 diabetic for almost 40 years. She lives in Manhattan, where she exercises by walking her dog three times a day and by gardening, which permit her to indulge in her favorite treat—very dark chocolate (in small-but-tasty quantities).

Don't miss these other titles from Bottom Line books and newsletters

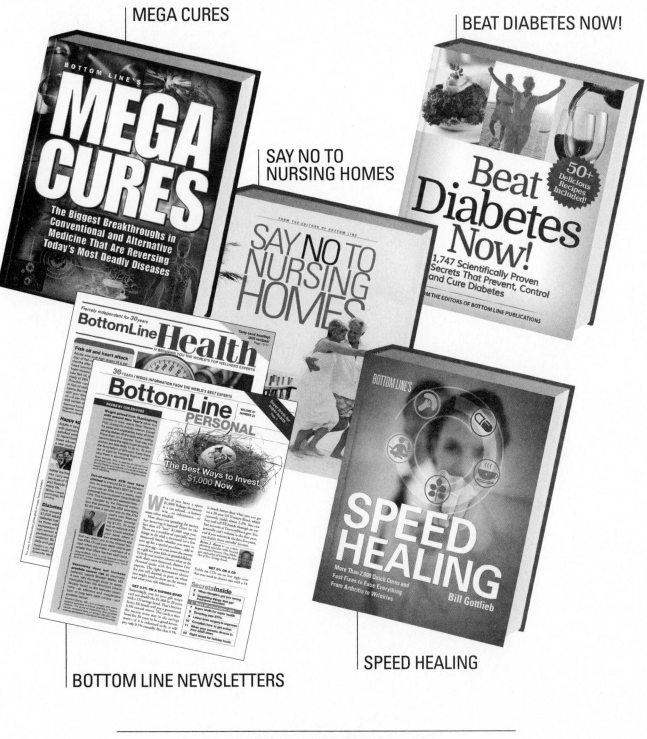

MEGA CURES

SAY NO TO NURSING HOMES

BEAT DIABETES NOW!

BOTTOM LINE NEWSLETTERS

SPEED HEALING

SHOP NOW FOR THE LATEST BREAKTHROUGHS

BOTTOMLINESTORE.COM